Congenital Spine Malformations

Khaled Fares AlAli • Hashim Talib Hashim
Editors

Congenital Spine Malformations

Clinical and Surgical Aspects

Springer

Editors
Khaled Fares AlAli
Department of Neurosurgery
Zayed Military Hospital, Abu Dhabi
Abu Dhabi, United Arab Emirates

Hashim Talib Hashim
Department of Research
University of Warith Al-Anbiyaa, College of Medicine
Karbala, Iraq

ISBN 978-3-031-59033-7 ISBN 978-3-031-59031-3 (eBook)
https://doi.org/10.1007/978-3-031-59031-3

This Springer imprint is published by the registered company Springer Nature Switzerland AG
The registered company address is: Gewerbestrasse 11, 6330 Cham, Switzerland

Paper in this product is recyclable.

Contents

Contributors

Mahdi Abdalhusain University of Malta, Msida, Malta

Zubia Afzal King Edward Medical University, Lahore, Pakistan

Yasmin Ahmadi School of Medicine, Royal College of Surgeons in Ireland-Bahrain, Busaiteen, Bahrain

Kani Ahmed School of Medicine, University of Sulaimani, Sulaymaniyah, Iraq

Hafiza Qurat Ul Ain CMH Multan Institute of Medical Sciences, Multan, Pakistan

Narjiss Aji Faculty of Medicine and Pharmacy of Rabat, Rabat, Morocco

K. G. Akashnath School of Medicine, Royal College of Surgeons in Ireland-Bahrain, Busaiteen, Bahrain

Usama AlDallal School of Medicine, Royal College of Surgeons in Ireland-Bahrain, Busaiteen, Bahrain

Mohammedbaqer Ali Al-Ghuraibawi Faculty of Medicine, University of Warith Al-Anbiyaa, Karbala, Iraq

Zainab A. Alkhuzaie College of Medicine, University of Kufa, Najaf, Iraq

Yasser F. Almealawy College of Medicine, University of Kufa, Najaf, Iraq

Ahmed Dheyaa Al-Obaidi College of Medicine, University of Baghdad, Baghdad, Iraq

Mustafa Najah Al-Obaidi College of Medicine, University of Baghdad, Baghdad, Iraq

Mohammed H. Al-Rammahi Department of Neurosurgery, 2021 Graduate of College of Medicine, University of Kufa, Najaf, Iraq

Abdullah Alsayedomar University of Malta, Msida, Malta

Zainab Aljameel Saad Al-Shami Faculty of Medicine, University of Warith Al-Anbiyaa, Karbala, Iraq

Leen Rikan Azzam School of Medicine, Royal College of Surgeons in Ireland-Bahrain, Busaiteen, Bahrain

Rebecca Caruana Department of Medicine and Surgery, University of Malta, Msida, Malta

Sage Ishimwe Marie Consolatrice School of Medicine, University of Global Health Equity, Butaro, Rwanda

Motaz Daraghma Faculty of Medicine, Arab American University of Palestine, Jenin, Palestine

Yazan Demaidi Department of Medicine, An-Najah National University, Nablus, Palestine

Sewar Elejla Al-Azhar University Gaza, Gaza, Palestine

Ahmed Mostafa Abd-Elhady Elhagar GP, Fayoum University Hospital, Fayoum, Egypt

Ahmed Elnahhas Faculty of medicine, Tanta University, Tanta, Egypt

Mohamed Osama Farouk Faculty of Medicine, Ain Shams University, Cairo, Egypt

Abdul Rehman Gull King Edward Medical University, Lahore, Pakistan

Yasir Khaleel Hameed College of Medicine, University of Baghdad, Baghdad, Iraq

Ghazwan Abdulla Hasan Royal Private Hospital, Baghdad, Iraq

Zeinab Yousef Hashem GP, Fayoum University Hospital, Fayoum, Egypt

Vanya Ibrahim Jwamer School of Medicine, University of Sulaimani, Sulaymaniyah, Iraq

Fatimah Dheyaa Kadhim College of Medicine, University of Kufa, Najaf, Iraq

Ateeba Kamran Karachi Medical and Dental College, Karachi, Pakistan

Ahmed Kazerooni College of Medicine and Medical Sciences, Arabian Gulf University, Manama, Bahrain

Umniah Khajori College of Medicine, University of Baghdad, Baghdad, Iraq

Sarah Zuhair Kurdi Kufa University-College of Medicine, Al-Sader Medical City, Najaf, Iraq

Emry Atwa Ibrahim Mansour Faculty of Medicine, Ain Shams University, Cairo, Egypt

Qasim Mehmood King Edward Medical University, Lahore, Pakistan

Michaela Micallef Department of Medicine and Surgery, University of Malta, Msida, Malta

Ahmed Ameer Mohammed Sulaiman Alrajhi University, Al Bukayriyah, Saudi Arabia

Tabarak Qassim School of Medicine, Royal College of Surgeons in Ireland-Bahrain, Busaiteen, Bahrain

Ahmed Hassan A. Rady Faculty of Medicine, Ain Shams University, Cairo, Egypt

Farhan Rana School of Medicine, Royal College of Surgeons in Ireland-Bahrain, Busaiteen, Bahrain

Ahmad Rjoub Department of Medicine, An-Najah National University, Nablus, Palestine

Mohamad Abdulwahab Sabsabee Sulaiman Alrajhi University, Al Bukayriyah, Saudi Arabia

Maryam Salman School of Medicine, Royal College of Surgeons in Ireland-Bahrain, Busaiteen, Bahrain

Natnael Shimelash School of Medicine, University of Global Health Equity, Butaro, Rwanda

Ahmed Talaia Faculty of Medicine, Tanta University, Tanta, Egypt

Jaafar I. Twayej Department of Medicine, 2022 Graduate of College of Medicine, University of Kufa, Najaf, Iraq

Theogene Uwizeyimana School of Medicine, University of Global Health Equity, Butaro, Rwanda

Ali Tarik Abdul Wahid Neurosurgery, Department of Surgery, College of Medicine, University of Baghdad, Baghdad, Iraq

Nael Wajdi College of Medicine, University of Baghdad, Baghdad, Iraq

Naseem Wajdi College of Medicine, University of Baghdad, Baghdad, Iraq

Chapter 1
General Introduction to Congenital Spine Malformations

Mohammedbaqer Ali Al-Ghuraibawi and Zainab Aljameel Saad Al-Shami

Spinal dysraphism represents a wide range of congenital anomalies that are mainly derived from a defect in the developmental process of the neural tube during the embryological period [1–3].

Generally, congenital spinal malformations are not rare and you can see many cases during your career [4]. As a neurosurgeon, being well aware of these malformations is very important to commit to a proper approach with better outcomes [5]. Depending on a specific anatomical or pathophysiological malformation congenital lesion, the symptoms could appear including motor and sensory pathways, bladder and bowel dysfunction, and deformity of bones [6–8]. Usually, it is necessary to correct these anomalies by surgical intervention to address the defect and limit its development [9–11]. Furthermore, these deformities can be associated with other anomalies such as hydrocephalus and Chiari II malformation, necessitating proper

M. A. Al-Ghuraibawi (✉) · Z. A. S. Al-Shami
Faculty of Medicine, University of Warith Al-Anbiyaa, Karbala, Iraq

K. F. AlAli, H. T. Hashim (eds.), *Congenital Spine Malformations*,
https://doi.org/10.1007/978-3-031-59031-3_1

assessment and treatment [12–15]. Mainly, congenital spinal malformations are classified into two main categories: spina bifida Aperta and spina bifida occulta. The first category (spina bifida Aperta) includes myelomeningocele, meningocele, or myeloschisis [16]. The other category (spina bifida occulta) involves lesions that are covered by skin (dermis and epidermis layers) such as split cord malformations, neuromeric cysts, lipoma, dermoid cysts, and lipo-myelomeningocele [17]. In the USA the incidence of these anomalies is about 1 per 1000 pregnancies. Folic acid supplements and maternal health have shown a decrease rate of neural tube worldwide. Nowadays, significant improvement is conducted to improve surgical and non-surgical technologies to treat and prevent these conditions [18].

Neurulation is the process of neural tube formation. The severity of deformity depends on this phase of embryological development which begins at day 18 of gestation. This is followed by the formation of the groove in the midline surrounded by neural folds on each side. The folds fuse dorsally, starting from the middle and extending in both the cranial and caudal directions [18–20]. Then the neural tube is formed, and after that, the neuropores (formation of the opening on each side) take place, these openings are closed on day 26. On the dorsal surface, the separation of the tube from the ectoderm occurs, and eventually, the ectoderm becomes the dermis and epidermis [21]. In the second phase of neurulation (secondary neurulation), the most caudal part of the neural tube develops from caudal cell masses produced by a regressing tail bud [22, 23]. Regression of the tail structure results in leaving behind the filum terminale, the coccygeal ligament, and the terminal ventricle of the conus. Spinal cord malformation will strongly depend on whether it occurred pre-neurulation or post-neurulation.

Spina bifida Aperta: Spina bifida is of several types, this condition may present in various forms, including open spina bifida (spina bifida cystica, myelomeningocele, and meningocele), closed spina bifida (lipo-myelomeningocele, and diastematomyelia).

Myelomeningocele (Meningomyelocele): The most common among all types of cystic spinal bifida, that is characterized by that the cyst contains nerves and parts from the spinal cord in plus tissue and cerebrospinal fluid (CSF). During pregnancy, the development of the spinal cord is damaged by fluid in the uterus, which leads to this defect [24]. This damage results almost always in paralysis and sensation loss, furthermore, the nerves to and from the cord are impacted [25].

Meningocele: Less common than other cystic types of spina bifida and usually causes less severe development impairment than other types. It is characterized by the sac doesn't contain spinal tissue, but it contains meninges and cerebrospinal fluid (CSF).

Spina bifida occulta (SBO): When there is one or more than one vertebrae are not closed completely. This form of spina bifida is covered by skin and it includes many specific conditions such as lipo-myelomeningocele, tethered cord, or diastematomyelia [26]. Each specific type requires a different approach to treatment, so it is very important to distinguish between each type.

Lipomyelomeningocoele: It is known as a congenital spinal cord disorder mainly is caused by the entanglement of a benign fatty tumor with part of the spinal cord and nerves [27]. Lip-myelomeningocele could develop during the period of early stages of pregnancy as a result of a failure of the neural tube closure, and its exact cause is still uncertain. The fatty tissue attaches to the spinal cord when the layer of the skin detaches from the neural tissue early, which leads to leaving the spina bifida gap. This gap could prevent the spinal bones from completely closing, resulting in a skin-covered lump on the baby's back at birth, which can vary in size, shape, and location. Most majority of those affected by lipomyelomeningocele exhibit markers at the site of the lesion such as fatty lumps, deep dimples, or birthmarks, which is an indication for the presentation of this condition [28].

Diastematomyelia: Is a congenital disorder that hampers the development of the spinal cord. Diastematomyelia is characterized by a split in the spinal cord into two longitudinal halves, usually in the lumbar region. The split can occur due to an additional piece of bone or a band of fibrous tissue, which may also lead to diplomyelia. The presence of the extra bone or tissue can cause the spinal cord to become tethered, which in turn can lead to a range of symptoms such as back pain, muscle weakness, and dysfunction of the bowel or bladder [29].

Treatment for diastematomyelia is detethering, which includes the removal of the additional bone or tissue aiming to spinal cord free [29, 30]. However, individuals without additional bone or tissue may only experience symptoms if the cord becomes tethered. In some cases, diastematomyelia may coexist with lipomyelomeningocele, a type of neural tube defect marked by the spinal cord and its covering protruding through a defect in the vertebral column [31, 32].

These conditions can be associated with a wide range of symptoms which presents depending on the exact site of lesion and physiological changes [33]. Symptoms include weakness, bladder and bowel dysfunction, hydrocephalus, and other associated complications may present [34].

Treatment or management approach will depend on the type of congenital abnormality and it differs from one patient to another [35]. Most of these malformations can be prevented by taking a supplement of folic acid or food that contains it in a sufficient amount [36, 37].

All details of the signs and symptoms of congenital spinal anomalies will be discussed in this textbook.

Multiple Choice Questions

1. **Regarding congenital scoliosis, which of the following is false:**

   A. The most common cause of congenital scoliosis is hemivertebra.
   B. Spinal deformity is based on two factors; vertebral level and the degree of segmentation.
   C. Severe progressive congenital scoliosis surgery is not an effective treatment.
   D. The most severe congenital deformities may result from a unilateral unsegmented bar.

2. **Myelomeningocele differs from the rest of the spinal dystrophic disorder in:**
   A. This happens due to an impairment of secondary neurulation.
   B. Occurs during the sixth gestational week.
   C. Being a pan-CNS disorder.
   D. Hydrocephalus is rarely reported in cases of myelomeningocele.
3. **All of these spinal dysraphisms occur during primary neurulation except:**
   A. Congenital dermal sinus.
   B. Split cord malformation.
   C. Filum terminal disorders.
   D. Lipomas.
4. **Regarding surgical treatment of neural tube defect:**
   A. Surgical treatment is mainly based on myelomeningocele closure.
   B. Asymptomatic NTD may just be followed up.
   C. Symptomatic NTD should undergo surgery as early as possible with intra-operative neurophysiological monitoring.
   D. Prophylactic correction of spinal lipomas is necessary.
5. **Which of the following is believed to be associated with gestational diabetes complications:**
   A. Caudal regression syndrome.
   B. Split cord malformation.
   C. Filum terminal disorders.
   D. Myelocele.
6. **Regarding congenital kyphosis, which of the following causes is wrong:**
   A. Failure of formation of the vertebral body.
   B. Failure of segmentation of the vertebral body.
   C. Mixed failure of formation and segmentation.
   D. Degeneration of the vertebral body.
7. **Regarding the types of congenital kyphosis, which of the following is true:**
   A. Type 1 (failure of formation of vertebral body).
   B. Type 2 (failure of segmentation with ventral unsegmented bar).
   C. Type 2 produces less deformity and is less likely to result in neuralgic defects.
   D. Type 1 produces severe deformity and neurologic defects.
8. **Initial treatment of dysplastic spondylolisthesis should be:**
   A. Now operative.
   B. Now operative unless there has been documented progression in young patients.
   C. Now operative unless there has been slippage of less than 50%.
   D. Surgical treatment is associated with less risk.

9. **All of these are true regarding lipo-myelomeningocele except:**
   A. The most common symptoms are bowel, and bladder symptoms, and progressive paralysis.
   B. Neurologic examination is usually abnormal at birth.
   C. The primary surgical aim is to untether the spinal cord.
   D. The mass covered by skin and the lipomatous tissue extends intradermally with the rootlets of cauda equina.

10. **The condition in which the spinal cord is bifid and the two hemi-cords are separated by bony spur is called:**
   A. Dermoid tumor.
   B. Diastematomyelia.
   C. Meningocele.
   D. Lipo-myelomeningocele.

References

1. Botto LD, Moore CA, Khoury MJ, Erickson JD. Neural-tube defects. N Engl J Med. 1999;341(20):1509–19.
2. Greene NDE, Copp AJ. Neural tube defects. Annu Rev Neurosci. 2014;37:221–42.
3. Thunem NY, Lowry RB, Tucker BJ, Medd BW. Birth prevalence and recurrence rates of neural tube defects in southern Alberta in 1970-81. CMAJ (Can Med Assoc J). 1988;138(9):819–23.
4. Williams J, Mai CT, Mulinare J, et al. Updated estimates of neural tube defects prevented by mandatory folic acid fortification—United States, 1995–2011. MMWR Morb Mortal Wkly Rep. 2015;64(1):1–5.
5. Copp AJ, Greene NDE. Neural tube defects—disorders of neurulation and related embryonic processes. Wiley Interdiscip Rev Dev Biol. 2013;2(2):213–27.
6. Moore K, Persaud TVN, Torchia M. Before we are born: essentials of embryology and birth defects. 8th ed. Philadelphia, PA: Elsevier; 2011.
7. Nakatsu T, Uwabe C, Shiota K. Neural tube closure in humans initiates at multiple sites: evidence from human embryos and implications for the pathogenesis of neural tube defects. Anat Embryol (Berl). 2000;201(6):455–66.
8. Copp AJ, Brook FA. Does lumbosacral spina bifida arise by failure of neural folding or by defective canalisation? J Med Genet. 1989;26(3):160–6.
9. Morioka T, Hashiguchi K, Mukae N, Sayama T, Sasaki T. Neurosurgical management of patients with lumbosacral myeloschisis. Neurol Med Chir (Tokyo). 2010;50(9):870–6.
10. Northrup H, Volcik KA. Spina bifida and other neural tube defects. Curr Probl Pediatr. 2000;30(10):313–32.
11. Sepulveda W, Wong AE, Sepulveda F, Alcalde JL, Devoto JC, Otayza F. Prenatal diagnosis of spina bifida: from intracranial translucency to intrauterine surgery. Childs Nerv Syst. 2017;33(7):1083–99.
12. Murakami N, Morioka T, Suzuki SO, et al. Clinicopathological findings of limited dorsal myeloschisis associated with spinal lipoma of dorsal-type. Interdiscip Neurosurg. 2020;21:100781. [Epub ahead of print]
13. Meadows JT Jr, Hayes D Jr. Rachischisis totalis without acrania in a newborn male. Pediatr Neurol. 2014;51(1):123–5.

14. Pang D, Zovickian J, Wong ST, Hou YJ, Moes GS. Limited dorsal myeloschisis: a not-so-rare form of primary neurulation defect. Childs Nerv Syst. 2013;29(9):1459–84.
15. Pang D, Zovickian J, Oviedo A, Moes GS. Limited dorsal myeloschisis: a distinctive clinico-pathological entity. Neurosurgery. 2010;67(6):1555–80.
16. Izci Y, Kural C. Limited dorsal myeloschisis with and without type I split cord malformation: report of 3 cases and surgical nuances. Medicine (Kaunas). 2019;55(2):28.
17. Morioka T, Suzuki SO, Murakami N, et al. Neurosurgical pathology of limited dorsal myeloschisis. Childs Nerv Syst. 2018;34(2):293–303.
18. Urui S, Oi S. Experimental study of the embryogenesis of open spinal dysraphism. Neurosurg Clin North Am. 1995;6(2):195–202.
19. Dias MS, Walker ML. The embryogenesis of complex dysraphic malformations: a disorder of gastrulation? Pediatr Neurosurg. 1992;18(5–6):229–53.
20. Elgamal EA. Natural history of hydrocephalus in children with spinal open neural tube defect. Surg Neurol Int. 2012;3:112.
21. Cleland. Contribution to the study of spina bifida, encephalocele, and anencephalus. J Anat Physiol. 1883;17(Pt 3):257–92.
22. McLone DG, Knepper PA. The cause of Chiari II malformation: a unified theory. Pediatr Neurosci. 1989;15(1):1–12.
23. Hahn YS. Open myelomeningocele. Neurosurg Clin N Am. 1995;6(2):231–41.
24. Pang D. Surgical complications of open spinal dysraphism. Neurosurg Clin N Am. 1995;6(2):243–57.
25. Babcook CJ. Ultrasound evaluation of prenatal and neonatal spina bifida. Neurosurg Clin N Am. 1995;6(2):203–18.
26. Apkon SD, Grady R, Hart S, et al. Advances in the care of children with spina bifida. Adv Pediatr Infect Dis. 2014;61(1):33–74.
27. North T, Cheong A, Steinbok P, Radic JA. Trends in incidence and long-term outcomes of myelomeningocele in British Columbia. Childs Nerv Syst. 2018;34(4):717–24.
28. Phillips LA, Burton JM, Evans SH. Spina bifida management. Curr Probl Pediatr Adolesc Health Care. 2017;47(7):173–7.
29. Begeerl JH, Meihuizen de Regt MJ, HogenEsch I, Ter Weeme CA, Mooij JJ, Vencken LM. Progressive neurological deficit in children with spina bifida aperta. Z Kinderchir. 1986;41(suppl 1):13–5.
30. McLone DG. Technique for closure of myelomeningocele. Childs Brain. 1980;6(2):65–73.
31. Moldenhauer JS, Adzick NS. Fetal surgery for myelomeningocele: after the management of Myelomeningocele Study (MOMS). Semin Fetal Neonatal Med. 2017;22(6):360–6.
32. Adzick NS, Thom EA, Spong CY, et al. A randomized trial of pre- natal versus postnatal repair of myelomeningocele. N Engl J Med. 2011;364(11):993–1004.
33. Brock 3rd JW, Carr MC, Adzick NS, etal. Bladderfunctionafterfetal surgery for myelomeningocele. Pediatrics. 2015;136(4):e906–e913
34. Farmer DL, Thom EA, Brock JW 3rd, et al. The management of myelomeningocele study: full cohort 30-month pediatric outcomes. Am J Obstet Gynecol. 2018;218(2):256.e1–256.e13.
35. Chan YY, Sandlin SK, Kurzrock EA. Urological outcomes of myelo- meningocele and lipomeningocele. Curr Urol Rep. 2017;18(5):35.
36. McLone DG. Continuing concepts in the management of spina bifida. Pediatr Neurosurg. 1992;18(5–6):254–6.
37. Bowman RM, McLone DG, Grant JA, Tomita T, Ito JA. Spina bifida outcome: a 25-year prospective. Pediatr Neurosurg. 2001;34(3):114–20.

Chapter 2
Epidemiology of Congenital Spine Malformation

Michaela Micallef, Rebecca Caruana, and Mustafa Najah Al-Obaidi

Test your learning and check your understanding of this book's contents: use the "Springer Nature Flashcards" app to access questions using ▶ https://sn.pub/QCsfpd.
To use the app, please follow the instructions in Chap. 1.

2.1 Introduction

Congenital spinal malformations (CSM) occur in a wide range of clinical presentations and can vary from mild to severe. In this chapter we will be tackling the epidemiology of various congenital spinal malformations including Spina bifida; Klippel Feil syndrome Congenital Scoliosis; Congenital kyphosis and Congenital lordosis;

CSM are inborn deformities of the vertebrae or neural tube which arise from abnormal spinal development during embryogenesis (i.e. in the first 8 weeks of life). Approximately 12% of the general population possess minor vertebral malformations which are often asymptomatic and only recognized on the routine lumbar spine or chest x-rays. Contrarily more consequential malformations which result in progressive spinal abnormalities occur at a prevalence of 0.5/1000 live births [1]. Spina bifida is also part of the CSM but results from a neural tube defect, rather than abnormalities in the vertebrae bodies as results in the other CSM [2].

M. Micallef (✉) · R. Caruana
Department of Medicine and Surgery, University of Malta, Msida, Malta
e-mail: michaela.m.micallef.18@um.edu.mt

M. N. Al-Obaidi
College of Medicine, University of Baghdad, Baghdad, Iraq

K. F. AlAli, H. T. Hashim (eds.), *Congenital Spine Malformations*,
https://doi.org/10.1007/978-3-031-59031-3_2

2.2 Spina Bifida

Spina Bifida is one of the most common congenital abnormalities, resulting from neural tube defects originating during embryogenesis day 18–20 [3]. SB is classified into 3 subtypes: spina bifida occulta, meningocele and myelomeningocele [4]. Recent studies have identified that the incidence rate of SB worldwide is 18.6 per 10,000 live births and an incident rate of 3.63 per 10,000 live births in the US. Higher rates of incidence have been linked with individuals residing in England, Wales, northern China and the eastern seaboard of the United States [5]. SB is more prevalent in Hispanics rather than non-Hispanic white mothers [6]. It has been identified that an estimated 220,000 neonates born worldwide annually have a neural tube defect, the highest % being in developing countries as a consequence of malnutrition [7]. Since the establishment of mandatory folic acid fortification in the US, as shown in a case study carried out on 2593 cases, the case severity has decreased by 70% which was most significant in non-Hispanic white mothers and the prevalence rate since the fortification in 1998–2016 has decreased by 23% [8]. A systematic review and meta-analysis of 20 studies with a total population of over 20 million live births and approximately 12,000 Spina Bifida infants showed a significant decline of 4.76% in infant mortality rate per 100,000 live births per year. This decline in severity and mortality rate can be attributed to mandatory folic acid food fortification, early detection and advances in spina bifida treatment [9]. SB can span from mild to severe, having minor disabilities to serious impairments. Depending on the severity, SB may be accompanied by bowel and/or bowel dysfunction, motor impairment and neurological sequestration. SB is also associated with Arnold-Chiari II malformations [10].

The etiology of SB is multifactorial having both genetic and environmental risk factors. The genetic component contributes to approximately 60–70%, with the identification of approximately 250 genes which result in neural tube defects [10]. There are many environmental risk factors ranging from medication such as (methotrexate, rifampin and valproate as these influence the folate metabolism), a diet with low folic acid, maternal diabetes mellitus, tobacco smoking, obesity, hyperthermia and environmental pollutants. To reduce the incidence of SB center of disease control and prevention incentivize women who are of childbearing age intake 400 mcg of folic acid per day and women who have a previous history of neural tube defect to consume 4000 mcg of folic acid daily [4].

2.3 Klippel Feil Syndrome

Klippel Feil syndrome (KFS) is a rare CSM, presenting with the congenital fusion of all or some of the cervical vertebrae, occurring from faulty cervical segmentation during early embryonic development at 3–8 weeks of gestation [11]. In spite of the clinical trial of diagnosis being (short neck, limited neck movement and low posterior hairline) studies have identified that only 40–50% display this clinical triad [2].

KFS has a prevalence rate of 1/40,000 live births globally, which is a higher incidence in females than in males with 60% of the affected patients being female [12]. Recently in a computed tomography-based analysis of 2917 patients, it was found that the prevalence of KFS was higher than previously reported with a prevalence of 1 in 172 live births. This was based on the reality that clinical diagnosis is not always fully dependent and most cases were identified fortuitously in imaging [13]. Three subtypes of KFS exist type 1 (massive cervical fusion, which may include the upper thoracic vertebrae), type 2 (fusion of one or two vertebrae and other associated abnormalities of the cervical spine) and type 3 (fusion of the cervical vertebrae with the associated fusion of the lower thoracic or lumbar vertebrae) [2]. In a study by [14] carried out on 22 patients with KFS, it was found that 54.5% were type 1, 27.3% were type 2 and 18.2% were type 3. While in a more recent study carried out by [15] on 28 patients, it was found that type 2 was most common (50%) with both type 2 and 3 beings (25%). In this study, it was also found that type 3 has a higher prevalence in males while type 1 has the highest prevalence in females and type 2 showed a similar prevalence in both sexes. It has been reported that C5–C6 and C2–C3 are the most commonly fused cervical vertebrae [13]. KFS presents from birth, but mild cases may be not recognized till later in life when symptoms first present or worsen. Approximate 50% of pediatric patients are symptomatic [15]. KFS patients as a result of the cervical anomalies result in conditions such as spondylosis 42%, cervical disc degeneration (100%), disc herniation (72.2%) and osteophyte formation (18.2%) as reported in studies carried out by Ulmer et al. and Guille et al. which may lead to the development of neurological sequence in the form of radiculopathy, myelopathy or paraplegia. In some clinical reviews carried out by [15] as mentioned above it was found that the average age for the development of cervical spine symptoms was 11.9 years. 36% of patients developed cervical spine symptoms, with type 1 being highly associated with axial neck symptoms, while type 2–3 patients were predominantly associated with radicular and myelopathic symptoms. Myelopathic patients developed cervical symptoms earliest with an average age of 10.6, then axial (13 years) and finally idiopathic symptoms (18.6 years).

KFS is also associated with a significant spectrum of associated anomalies such as scoliosis in 60% of cases being worst in in type 1 and decreases in severity in type 2 and 3, respectively [2], renal anomalies in 35–55%, spina bifida occulta in 45%, congenital heart defects in 8–14%, hearing impairment in 30–40%, rib abnormalities in 20–30%, synkinesis in 20%, Sprengel anomaly in 20–30% [16]. Other infrequent anomalies include: ear deformities, intestinal anomalies, craniofacial abnormalities and congenital limb deformities [11].

2.4 Congenital Scoliosis

Congenital scoliosis (CS) is the most frequent spinal malformation [17]. CSM is a CSM resulting in lateral curvature of the spine, arising from anomalies occurring during embryogenic vertebral development caused by failure of formation and/or segmentation of the vertebrae or a combination of both. The worldwide prevalence of CS is 0.5–1/1000 live births [18], with a slightly higher rate in females than in males, with a ratio of 1.4:1. A study conducted from a nationwide health insurance database (2010–2015) showed that over a 5-year period the incidence rate of CS was 3.08 per 100,000 persons, with the highest incidence being at 0 years and the second highest at 12–16 years. CS presents at birth, but clinical deformity may not be evident until later in childhood when progressive scoliosis becomes perceptible. CS tends to progress quickly during the preadolescent growth spurt approximately after 10 years of age [19]. It was identified that 25% of CS cases were remarkably progressive, 50% were moderately progressive and the remaining 25% were non-progressive [20]. Most patients with congenital scoliosis will require a form of surgical intervention. Studies have shown that the postoperative mortality and morbidity of paediatric scoliosis surgery range from (0.12%–0.17%) and (3.7%–14.9%), respectively [21].

CS is closely linked with other malformations, having approximately 4–7 other different organ malformations, which range in location from (25%) genitourinary anomalies, (10%–15%) cardiac anomalies and also (28%–40%) spinal dysraphism (e.g intradural lipoma, diastematomyelia, fibrous dural band, syringomyelia, or tethered spinal cord). Other anomalies which may be associated include Goldenhar syndrome (oculoauriculovertebral dysplasia), Sprengel deformity, anal atresia, Klippel-Feil, CHARGE and VACTERL syndrome [18, 22].

The etiology of CS is multifactorial and can be divided into both genetic and environmental risk factors. The genetic link has been established from the presence of CS occurring with other vertebral anomalies resulting in a 5–10% increased risk of another sibling having vertebral anomalies [18]. The genetics are still not fully understood but these genes have been linked with the development of CS and other CSM: null mutation and a hypomorphic allele of the T-box 6 (TBX6) gene accountable for 10% sporadic CS [23], LFNG mutation [24], and FBN1 gene mutation. On the other hand, Environmental risk factors which may play a role in the pathogenesis of CS include hypoxia, Gestational Diabetes, carbon monoxide exposure from cigarette smoking, hyperthermia, alcohol, drugs such as valproic acid and environmental toxins such as boric acid [18]. Reducing exposure to such environmental factors may reduce the risk of simultaneous CS.

2.5 Congenital Kyphosis

Congenital kyphosis (CK) originates from defects of anterior formation (type 1) or segmentation (type 2) or from a combination of both defects (type 3), in one or more of the vertebrae in the sagittal plane during the first few weeks of embryonic development. This results in the progressive formation of a sharp forward curve (kyphosis) as the individual grows older [25]. The precise incidence of CK is unknown, however, the expected rates are approximately 3–4/10,000 live birth [26]. In spite of CK being congenital it is not always visible from birth, type 1 is visible from birth and worsens with growth while type 2 is more likely to be missed at birth and be identified as the child starts ambulating [27]. In the early stages of type 2 CK, it is relatively hard to differentiate CK from Scheuermann disease, in which the vertebrae grow unevenly resulting in hyperkyphosis. Scheuermann disease has a prevalence rate of 1–8% in the United States, occurring most commonly in males (2:1) and is diagnosed most commonly at the age of >12 [28]. Unfortunately, CK tends to aggravate with age and about 18–25% of patients result in neurological defects such as paraplegia and spinal cord compression [25]. Without any surgical intervention and treatment CK most often progresses thus surgery should be carried out at the earliest convenience ideally before the age of 5, before the kyphosis exceeds more than 50 ° [29]. CK like CS may present with other anomalies such as cardiac and renal anomalies as they form during the same embryonic period [27]. The precedes aetiology of CK is not known and is believed to be caused by a vascularization disorder as animal studies suggest [30].

2.6 Congenital Lordosis

Congenital lordosis (CL) is a rare CSM which originates from a defect in posterior segmentation during embryological development resulting in an excessive inward curvature of the spine[2]. The exact prevalence and incidence of CL are unknown however a systematic review and meta-analysis of 6 studies done on school-age children (7–15 years) in Iran with a population of 29,758, revealed that the prevalence rate was 32.59% and lordosis was higher among girls 1.6:1 [31]. CL is progressive and if left untreated can result in severe lordosis which can lead to altered rib mechanism resulting in atelectasis and severe pulmonary distress which may eventually lead to death. CK like other CSM is often also associated with other anomalies such as genitourinary cardiac and nervous system malformations [2].

Multiple Choice Questions

1. **............... is one of the most common congenital abnormalities?**

   A. Spina bifida
   B. Caudal regression syndrome
   C. Encephalocele
   D. Spinal stenosis

2. **........................... is a rare CSM which originates from a defect in posterior segmentation during embryological development resulting in an excessive inward curvature of the spine?**

   A. Kyphosis
   B. Scoliosis
   C. Congenital lordosis (CL)
   D. Spina bifida

3. **The worldwide prevalence of CS is .... live births?**
   A. 3–4/1000
   B. 0.5–1/1000
   C. 0.5–0.9/1000
   D. 5/1000
4. **The genetic component contributes to approximately .... with the identification of approximately 250 genes which result in neural tube defects.**
   A. 70%
   B. 40%
   C. 20%
   D. 60–70%
5. **........... is closely linked with other malformations, having approximately 4–7 other different organ malformations.**
   A. Kyphosis
   B. Lordosis
   C. Congenital scoliosis
   D. Spina bifida

Answers
1. A
2. C
3. B
4. D
5. C

References

1. Brand MC. Examination of the newborn with congenital scoliosis: focus on the physical. Adv Neonatal Care. 2008;8:265–73.
2. Kaplan KM, Spivak JM, Bendo JA. Embryology of the spine and associated congenital abnormalities. Spine J. 2005;5:564–76.
3. Paschereit F, Schindelmann KH, Hummel M, Schneider J, Stoltenburg-Didinger G, Kaindl AM. Cerebral abnormalities in spina bifida: a neuropathological study. Paediatr Dev Pathol. 2022;25:107–23.
4. Gober J, Thomas SP, Gater DR. Paediatric spina bifida and spinal cord injury. J Pers Med. 2022;12:985.
5. Au KS, Ashley-Koch A, Northrup H. Epidemiologic and genetic aspects of spina bifida and other neural tube defects. Dev Disabil Res Rev. 2010;16:6–15.
6. Agopian AJ, Canfield MA, Olney RS, Lupo PJ, Ramadhani T, Mitchell LE, Shaw GM, Moore CA, National Birth Defects Prevention Study. Spina bifida subtypes and sub-phenotypes by maternal race/ethnicity in the National Birth Defects Prevention Study. Am J Med Genet A. 2012;158:109–15.
7. Kondo A, Matsuo T, Morota N, Kondo AS, Okai I, Fukuda H. Neural tube defects: risk factors and preventive measures. Congenit Anom. 2017;57:150–6.

8. Mai CT, Evans J, Alverson CJ, Yue X, Flood T, Arnold K, Nestoridi E, Denson L, Adisa O, Moore CA. Changes in spina bifida lesion level after folic acid fortification in the US. J Pediatr. 2022;249:59–66.e1.
9. Ho P, Quigley MA, Tatwavedi D, Britto C, Kurinczuk JJ. Neonatal and infant mortality associated with spina bifida: a systematic review and meta-analysis. PLoS One. 2021;16:e0250098.
10. Hassan AS, Du YL, Lee SY, Wang A, Farmer DL. Spina bifida: a review of the genetics, pathophysiology and emerging cellular therapies. J Dev Biol. 2022;10:22.
11. Frikha R. Klippel-Feil syndrome: a review of the literature. Clin Dysmorphol. 2020;29:35–7.
12. Pizzutillo PD, Woods M, Nicholson L, MacEwen GD. Risk factors in Klippel-Feil syndrome. Spine. 1994;19:2110–6.
13. Gruber J, Saleh A, Bakhsh W, Rubery PT, Mesfin A. The prevalence of Klippel-Feil syndrome: a computed tomography–based analysis of 2,917 patients. Spine Deform. 2018;6:448–53.
14. Guille JT, Miller A, Bowen JR, Forlin E, Caro PA. The natural history of Klippel-Feil syndrome: clinical, roentgenographic, and magnetic resonance imaging findings at adulthood. J Pediatr Orthop. 1995;15:617–26.
15. Samartzis D, Herman J, Lubicky JP, Shen FH. Classification of congenitally fused cervical patterns in Klippel-Feil patients: epidemiology and role in the development of cervical spine-related symptoms. Spine. 2006;31:E798–804.
16. Jcvankovičová A, Jakubíková J, Ďurovčíková D. A case of Klippel–Feil syndrome with congenital enlarged Eustachian tube. Int J Pediatr Otorhinolaryngol. 2012;76:596–600.
17. Pahys JM, Guille JT. What's new in congenital scoliosis? J Paediatr Orthop. 2018;38:e172–9.
18. Sebaaly A, Daher M, Salameh B, Ghoul A, George S, Roukoz S. Congenital scoliosis: a narrative review and proposal of a treatment algorithm. EFORT Open Rev. 2022;7:318–27.
19. Hedequist D, Emans J. Congenital scoliosis: a review and update. J Paediatr Orthop. 2007;27:106–16.
20. Cho W, Shepard N, Arlet V. The aetiology of congenital scoliosis: genetic vs. environmental—a report of three monozygotic twin cases. Eur Spine J. 2018;27:533–7.
21. Taniguchi Y, Oichi T, Ohya J, Chikuda H, Oshima Y, Matsubayashi Y, Matsui H, Fushimi K, Tanaka S, Yasunaga H. In-hospital mortality and morbidity of paediatric scoliosis surgery in Japan: analysis using a national inpatient database. Medicine. 2018;97:e0277.
22. Arlet V, Odent T, Aebi M. Congenital scoliosis. Eur Spine J. 2003;12:456–63.
23. Chen W, Lin J, Wang L, Li X, Zhao S, Liu J, Akdemir ZC, Zhao Y, Du R, Ye Y. TBX6 missense variants expand the mutational spectrum in a non-Mendelian inheritance disease. Hum Mutat. 2020;41:182–95.
24. Takeda K, Kou I, Mizumoto S, Yamada S, Kawakami N, Nakajima M, Otomo N, Ogura Y, Miyake N, Matsumoto N. Screening of known disease genes in congenital scoliosis. Mol Genet Genomic Med. 2018;6:966–74.
25. Xu H, Li C, Ma Z, Wu Z, Sha J, Diwu W, Yan Y, Liu Z, Fan Z, Huang L. Closing-opening wedge osteotomy for the treatment of congenital kyphosis in children. J Orthop Surg. 2022;30:10225536221118600.
26. McMaster MJ. Spinal growth and congenital deformity of the spine. Spine. 2006;31:2284–7.
27. Kale P, Dhawas A, Kale S, Tayade A, Thakre S. Congenital kyphosis in thoracic spine secondary to absence of two thoracic vertebral bodies. J Clin Diagn Res. 2015;9:TD03.
28. Mansfield JT, Bennett M. Scheuermann disease. 2018.
29. McMaster MJ, Singh H. The surgical management of congenital kyphosis and kyphoscoliosis. Spine. 2001;26:2146–54.
30. Audat ZA, Radaideh AM, Odat MA, Bashaireh KM, Mohaidat ZM, Assmairan MA, Alshbool OK, Audit NZ. Severe thoracolumbar congenital kyphosis treated with single posterior approach and gradual "in situ" correction. J Orthop Surg. 2020;28:2309499019898845.
31. Taleschian-Tabrizi N, Alinezhad F, Pezeshki MZ, Dastgiri S, Eftekharsadat B, Dolatkhah N. Prevalence of spinal deformities among school age children in Iran: a systematic review and meta-analysis. Int J Paediatr. 2022;10:16402–16.

Chapter 3
The Diagnosis of Congenital Spine Malformations

Qasim Mehmood, Hafiza Qurat Ul Ain, Abdul Rehman Gull, and Zubia Afzal

> Test your learning and check your understanding of this book's contents: use the "Springer Nature Flashcards" app to access questions using ▶ https://sn.pub/QCsfpd.
> To use the app, please follow the instructions in Chap. 1.

3.1 Introduction

Congenital spine abnormalities are spinal conditions that manifest in a person before birth. Early in fetal development, the vertebrae do not develop properly, which leads to structural issues with the spine and spinal cord [1]. The vertebrae are frequently absent, fused together, misshaped, or only partially developed in certain conditions. One or more congenital spine abnormalities may exist in an individual. Congenital spine abnormalities are caused by flaws that are currently unknown to medical researchers. Understanding congenital spine abnormalities' causes and how they affect the postnatal growing spine requires an understanding of the stages of the spine's development. The etiology of congenital spine abnormalities can be genetic, environmental, dietary, or a combination of multiple factors; however, in most cases, the underlying cause is unknown. Defective somitogenesis causes congenital spine abnormalities, which are linked to vitamin A deficiency (VAD).

Q. Mehmood (✉)
King Edward Medical University, Lahore, Pakistan

H. Q. U. Ain
CMH Multan Institute of Medical Sciences, Multan, Pakistan

A. R. Gull · Z. Afzal
King Edward Medical University, Lahore, Pakistan

K. F. AlAli, H. T. Hashim (eds.), *Congenital Spine Malformations*,
https://doi.org/10.1007/978-3-031-59031-3_3

However, little is known about the molecular pathways underlying congenital abnormalities linked to VAD [2, 3]. Preconception environmental factors, such as maternal obesity, poor nutrition, tobacco use, hyperhomocysteinemia, sedentarism, diabetes, and mental stress, play a central role in congenital spinal malformations, given their relation to excessive oxidative stress and inflammation, which speed up the telomerase shortening process that causes maternal biologic aging [4, 5].

3.2 Types of Congenital Spine Malformations

Congenital malformations of the spine can be scoliosis, lordoscoliosis, kyphoscoliosis, and pure kyphosis. These abnormalities develop when one or more vertebrae fail to develop symmetrically, causing a localized imbalance in the spine's longitudinal growth and a developing curvature that affects the coronal and/or sagittal planes with potential for advancement during skeletal development. The most prevalent congenital spine defect is congenital scoliosis. An abnormal lateral curving of the spine is known as scoliosis. Spinal curvature in the "coronal" (frontal) plane is a common definition of scoliosis. Scoliosis is a more complicated, three-dimensional issue that incorporates the coronal plane, sagittal plane, or axial plane; however, the coronal plane is where the degree of curvature is measured [6].

The second most common congenital anomaly is kyphosis. A genetic error that affects the formation or segmentation of the front portion of one or more vertebral bodies and discs takes place during the first 6–8 weeks of embryonic life. Congenital kyphosis can be classified into two categories: failure of segmentation and failure of formation. A kyphosis is caused by the failure of one or more vertebral bodies to form completely (Type I deformity), most commonly in the thoracolumbar spine. When two or more vertebrae fail to separate and create regular discs and rectangular bones, a deformity known as a failure of segmentation (Type II deformity) results. The diagnosis of this kind of congenital kyphosis is frequently made after the kid has begun walking. When there is a significant curve, the condition is also referred to as hunchback or round back [6].

Another congenital deformity is lordosis, which is the least common of the major congenital spinal deformities. The lumbar spine's aberrant inward curvature has historically been referred to as lordosis. It results from a posterior segmentation failure in the presence of anterior active growth [6].

3.3 Clinical Manifestations

The clinical manifestations of congenital anomalies of the spine vary. Some anomalies may be benign, resulting in no spinal deformity, and they may go unnoticed for the entirety of a person's life. However, some spinal defects do not manifest until later in childhood and/or adolescence, when symptoms deteriorate. Congenital spine abnormalities are sometimes manifested physically as a tilted pelvis, trouble breathing, aberrant back curvature or twisting to the left or right, forward or backward, or unequal shoulders, hips, waist, or legs [6, 7]. The selection of a diagnostic method that is specific to a patient (or case) is essential, so we should be familiar with their fundamental characteristics and methods. Before considering surgery for congenital spine deformities, nonoperative therapy is typically advised such as painkillers, physical therapy (which includes gait and posture training), and specific braces [7].

3.4 Prenatal Diagnosis

Prenatal screening of spina bifida and other congenital anomalies has become a prerequisite in all pregnancies. An anomaly scan is performed at 20 weeks to rule out these anomalies. There are other screening tests like alpha-fetoprotein assays and beta hCG to confirm the diagnosis early in pregnancy, however, the ultrasound scan has become the standard. Once confirmed, it is mandatory to undergo the required tests for the management and counseling of the patient.

Following tests can be performed for diagnosis and confirmation of spina bifida and other congenital spine malformations prenatally:

3.4.1 Laboratory Tests

Various laboratory tests can be performed for the diagnosis of congenital spine anomalies. Some of them are as follows:

Triple Screen Blood Test

This laboratory test is usually done in the second trimester (15–22 weeks) and looks for elevated AFP in the blood as it is a good indicator of the high risk of neural tube defects. The other two parts of this test are to look for human chorionic gonadotropin (hCG) and estriol. Inhibin A has also been included in this test, making it a quadruple test. The significance of this test is that AFP is made by the fetal liver, which also crosses the placenta and is present in maternal blood. The presence of this AFP in a pregnant woman can indicate several disease processes and requires proper investigation to rule out different causes. In spina bifida, AFP is present in unusually high amounts, especially in open neural tube defects, including spina bifida and anencephaly [8].

Amniocentesis

Amniotic fluid may also be tested for high levels of AFP and acetylcholinesterase as a confirmatory test after a triple screen during the 16th–20th weeks. Amniotic fluid analysis can also be done for chromosomal abnormalities, which may also result in high levels of AFP. Maternal serum alpha-fetoprotein (MS-AFP) was the first test to be used to diagnose open NTDs [8]. This was started after observing high levels of amniotic AFP in third-trimester pregnancies that were later found to end in babies with open defects [9]. Later, it was designed for women who had high MS-AFP (2.5 times the normal value) to undergo USG testing to exclude other causes of high AFP like incorrect gestational age, twin pregnancies, and fetal death [9].

3.4.2 Ultrasonography

Most pregnant females get their anomaly scan at 18–24 weeks of gestation. It has become a routine anomaly scan to rule out any congenital defects. It can be done earlier too if the blood screening tests or amniocentesis for AFP comes positive. The USG of the fetus can successfully detect spinal cord malformations as early as 11–14 weeks of gestation. An experienced sonographer can look at fetal nuchal translucency thickness, nasal bone length, and ductus venosus waveforms to detect anomalies. In a recent study, the biparietal diameter was used as a reference, with less than the fifth percentile seen in more than 50% of spina bifida patients [10]. A high-frequency transducer is required in ultrasound for accurate detection of neural tube involvement in NTDs. However, mostly 6–8 Hz transducers are commonly used for obstetric scans and can be used to detect early neural tube defects or abnormal limb positioning. 3D ultrasound facilities are even better for visualizing spinal anomalies, especially if 2D ultrasound is unable to fully show them [11].

Ultrasonography can help in differentiating between open and closed spina bifida as well. As both defects have different prognoses and require different management, it is important to differentiate between the two. The most common feature that separates the two is the cranial anatomy of the fetus. Open defects are more likely to have cranial signs like Arnold Chiari Malformation as compared to closed defects. Moreover, open defects are found to have increased levels of amniotic AFP and acetylcholinesterase [12]. There have been a number of features identified in first-trimester ultrasound scans that help in identifying open spina bifida [13], including the "lemon sign," which means the characteristic scalloping sign of the frontal bones due to tethering of the spine at the site of the spina bifida and subsequent downward displacement of the brain [14].

One of the suggested screening protocols is as follows.

1. MS-AFP less than 2 times the normal value requires no further action.
2. MS-AFP greater than 2 times the normal value requires an ultrasound to check the date of pregnancy.

3. If there is a difference of fewer than 10 days from the last menstrual period, screening is positive. If the difference is greater than 10 days but, after adjustment of MS-AFP according to the dates, is still more than twice the normal value, screening is still considered positive. For such cases, genetic counseling, risks, and benefits of amniocentesis and confirmatory ultrasound should be considered [15].

3.4.3 Magnetic Resonance Imaging (MRI)

Although MRI scans are not considered screening tests for the detection of spinal anomalies, prenatal MRI scans can better delineate the neural elements involved in neural tube defects [16]. These scans can help in deciding the future of pregnancy if termination is an option, in utero surgery for defects, and for planning delivery [17] With the ability to distinguish between closed NTDs and open NTDs, it is considered an efficient diagnostic test to determine the prognosis of defect, as closed NTD have a better prognosis with greater bladder function and lesser risk of scoliosis [14, 18]. MRI can be used to assess the location of the conus, and identify lipoma or other soft tissue masses within the spinal canal [17].

Usually, 1.5 or 3 Tesla fields are used for standard MRI tests. However, it cannot be used to detect syrinx, fatty filum, or the alignment of the spine [17]. Furthermore, fetal movements can challenge the imaging even in standard planes, but 2–4 mm thin sections can reduce the effects of fetal movement and provide better image quality [14, 16]. Other options are available, including fast pulse sequences such as steady-state free precession, half-Fourier acquisition single-shot turbo spin echo, fast T1-weighted gradient echo, and echo planar imaging. Gadolinium contrast agents cannot be used in pregnant women since gadolinium can cross the placenta and be toxic to the fetus [19].

3.5 Postnatal Diagnosis

If, for any reason, anomaly scans were not performed during pregnancy or any congenital spine defects went unnoticed, post-natal scans can prove to be beneficial to diagnose congenital spine malformations.

3.5.1 Clinical Examination

A baby born with a congenital spinal anomaly may have a different presentation according to the specific type. The congenital defect may be open or closed. The open defect may present in spina bifida aperta or myelomeningocele and meningocele; in these cases, skin over the defect does not form properly leading to the exposed spine or spinal nerves. Whereas, in a closed defect, the skin is covering the defect, which may even lead to difficulty in pointing out the defect, such as spina bifida occulta. Sometimes the defect is covered with a tuft of hair making it obvious [20].

Signs and symptoms may appear later in life and can cause one or more of the following:

- Pain and tenderness.
- Altered sensation including numbness and tingling.
- Altered motor function leading to difficulty in sitting or walking.
- Bowel and bladder problems (urinary incontinence, retention, constipation, etc.).
- Breathing difficulties in severe cases [20].

Spina bifida occulta may not present any symptoms and may be discovered incidentally on imaging tests for an unrelated reason. It may present as a tuft of hair, a dimple, or a birthmark. Meningocele is a simple collection of spinal fluid protruding through the skin and does not involve the nerves, therefore may present with bowel and bladder problems. Whereas myelomeningocele, a severe form of spina bifida, involves exposed nerves and membranes and may result in bowel and bladder dysfunction as well as a risk of life-threatening infections [20].

Bowel and bladder dysfunction is usually missed at the neonatal and infant stage and gets noticed later in life as patients may present with incontinence or inability to get toilet training, frequent urinary tract infections, etc. This may delay the diagnosis of spina bifida, especially in minor cases where no other signs or symptoms are present [21].

3.5.2 Plain Radiography

Closed neural tube defects, or spina bifida occulta, may present with a tuft of hair, dimple, or birthmark, so a simple X-ray of the spine can be diagnostic. Plain radiographs of the spine should be taken early in the post-natal period as it may help in detecting spinal anomalies which were noted or missed in prenatal scans. The optimum period is the first 2 months as vertebrae start to ossify after this period. Congenital vertebral anomalies may be associated with increased chances of spinal anomalies (around 15%). In some cases, spinal bifida occulta may be diagnosed accidentally due to a radiograph done for another reason [21].

3.5.3 Ultrasonography

An ultrasound performed during the 6th–12th week (before laminar ossification) can show intraspinal anomalies [21]. The spine is cartilaginous in neonates and infants; therefore, allow the ultrasound beam to pass and assess the spinal cord for any defects. Visualization of the spinal cord can be done in young children up to 12 years of age; however, the accuracy decreases with increasing age, over 5 months of age. Ultrasound is the preferred modality for diagnosing spinal cord anomalies over a CT scan or myelogram, as the latter options require sedation. Moreover, ultrasound is rapid, less expensive, and readily available [22].

The ultrasonographic features of the normal spinal cord and those of spinal anomalies have been discussed profusely. Ultrasonography can also aid in identifying lipomas as they are more echogenic compared to surrounding subcutaneous fat and neural tissue. It is generally believed that direct contact of the transducer with open defects should not be made, as it can damage the nerves and increase the chances of infection [22].

In the case of closed neural tube defects in a newborn, ultrasound is a particularly useful diagnostic modality due to its non-invasive nature. A tethered cord can be diagnosed by the sonographic features of the inability to visualize a normally tapered conus, a thickened filum terminale, a posteriorly located spinal cord within the spinal canal, a widened dural sac, and the absence of normal spinal cord rhythmic movements [22].

3.5.4 Magnetic Resonance Imaging (MRI)

MRI demonstrates neural elements better than other imaging modalities [23–25]. However, performing MRI with infant movements can prove to be a challenge, especially when anesthesia or sedation at such an early age can prove to have deleterious effects [26–28]. Therefore, the feed and wrap technique is used to obtain MRIs for infants to avoid anesthesia and heavy sedation. MRI is considered the second-line mode of diagnosing congenital spinal cord anomalies after ultrasound [29].

MRI can help in detecting several types and kinds of congenital spinal cord anomalies ranging from conus cysts to spina bifida and sacral/coccygeal agenesis [30]. MRI is specifically beneficial in differentiating open and closed neural tube defects. Although MRI is thought to be a better technique than CT myelogram, the latter can prove to be more beneficial and sensitive in identifying fibrous and neurovascular stalks making a diagnosis of diastematomyelia easier [31].

Even though MRI is one of the best imaging for the detection of neural involvement in NTDs but necessity of its use is debated. Therefore, it is generally used when the patient shows clinical signs of spinal anomalies or is undergoing spinal surgery. Otherwise, in case the anomaly is minor or it shows no clinical signs, MRI can be postponed to older age as it would be easier to perform or it may not be needed at all [17].

3.6 Conclusion

Congenital spine malformations are a group of anomalies that develop in children before their birth. When the vertebral column doesn't develop properly during fetal development in utero, it can cause structural as well as functional defects in the spine and spinal cord. The severity of these conditions ranges from mild deformities to life-threatening conditions. They can be diagnosed prenatally using blood tests, ultrasound scans, MRIs, and amniocentesis. Postnatally, clinical examination, X-ray, CT scan, or MRI can be used for their diagnosis.

Multiple Choice Questions

1. **In which week of embryogenesis, spine and cord start growing?**

   A. First week
   B. Second week
   C. Third week
   D. Fourth week
   E. None of the above

   Answer: A

   Explanation: Starting in the first weeks of gestation, the spine and spinal cord grow.

2. **Deficiency of which vitamin is linked to defective somatogenesis?**

   A. Vitamin D
   B. Vitamin C
   C. Vitamin A
   D. Vitamin B
   E. None of the above

   Answer: C

   Explanation: Defective somatogenesis causes congenital spine abnormalities, which are linked to vitamin A deficiency (VAD).

3. **Which one of the following is most prevalent congenital spinal deformity?**

   A. Kyphosis
   B. Scoliosis
   C. Lordosis
   D. None of the above

   Answer: B

   Explanation: The most prevalent congenital spine defect is congenital scoliosis.

4. **Congenital abnormalities result from the failure in the growth of spine in which plane?**

   A. Longitudinal plane
   B. Horizontal plane

C. Vertical plane
D. Both A and B
E. None of the above

Answer: A

Explanation: Congenital abnormalities develop when one or more vertebrae fail to develop symmetrically, causing a localized imbalance in the spine's longitudinal growth.

5. **Which one of the following is First line imaging in infants?**

A. CT scan
B. X-ray
C. MRI
D. Ultrasound
E. None of the above

Answer: D

Explanation: Because of their special characteristic of the still cartilaginous nature of the yet-unossified future bony structures of the vertebral spine, ultrasound (US) should be used as the first line imaging in neonates and young infants.

6. **The most important hormone in quadruple screening test for neural tube defects is:**

A. hCG
B. Estriol
C. AFP
D. Inhibin A
E. None of the above

Answer: C

Explanation: AFP is the most important hormone to detect in maternal serum or amniotic fluid during pregnancy to detect neural tube defects in the fetus.

7. **Anomaly scan is mostly done during**

A. 20–26 weeks of pregnancy
B. 18–24 weeks of pregnancy
C. 10–16 weeks of pregnancy
D. After birth
E. It is no longer done

Answer: B

Explanation: Most pregnant females undergo anomaly scan at 18–24 weeks of pregnancy.

8. **Arnold Chiari malformations are more likely to occur with**

A. Open NTDs
B. Closed NTDs
C. Both A and B

D. Neither A and B
E. Lower than normal AFP levels

Answer: A

Explanation: Arnold Chiari malformation is more likely to occur with open neural tube defects and raised AFP levels.

9. **"Lemon sign" in open spina bifida ultrasound scan of first trimester shows:**

A. Appearance of the cerebellum wrapped around the medulla
B. Appearance of the choroid plexuses on axial imaging
C. Characteristic scalloping sign of frontal bones
D. Posterior displacement and deformation of the mesencephalon
E. None of the above

Answer: C

Explanation: Lemon sign is seen in first trimester ultrasound scan of open spinal bifida as characteristic scalloping sign of frontal bones.

10. **Which of these investigations is considered gold standard investigation for neural tube defects?**

A. MRI
B. AFP levels
C. CT Scan
D. Ultrasound
E. None of the above

Answer: D

Explanation: Ultrasound is considered gold standard investigation for identifying neural tube defects in fetus.

11. **The spinal anomaly most commonly associated with a dimple, tuft of hair or birthmark is**

A. Myelomeningocele
B. Meningocele
C. Spina bifida occulta
D. Spina bifida aperta
E. None of these

Answer: C

Explanation: Spina bifida occulta is most common spinal anomaly to present with a dimple, birthmark or tuft of hair.

12. **Which of the following has the highest risk of bowel and bladder problems and life-threatening infections in the fetus?**

A. Spina bifida occulta
B. Meningocele
C. Tethered spine
D. Myelomeningocele
E. Both A and B

Answer: D

Explanation: Myelomeningocele has the highest risk of bowel and bladder problems and life-threatening infections as nerves of the spinal cord are exposed in this condition.

13. **A postnatal ultrasound to detect spinal anomalies is best to be done**

    A. At birth
    B. During 6th–12th week
    C. After 5 months
    D. At 2 years
    E. At 15 years

Answer: B

Explanation: A postnatal ultrasound to detect spinal anomalies is best to be done during 6th–12th week before laminar ossification.

14. **Imaging modality to best demonstrate the neural element involvement in spina bifida in infants is**

    A. Ultrasound
    B. CT scan
    C. MRI
    D. Both B and C
    E. Neither

Answer: C

Explanation: MRI demonstrates neural element better than other imaging modalities.

15. **A tethered cord can be diagnosed by sonographic features of**

    A. Inability to visualize normal tapered conus
    B. A thickened filum terminale
    C. Posteriorly located spinal cord within the spinal canal
    D. Absence of normal spinal cord rhythmic movements
    E. All of the above

Answer: E

Explanation: All of these sonographic features help in diagnosing tethered spinal cord.

References

1. Nabizadeh N, Dimar JR. Congenital spine deformities: timing of insult during development of the spine in utero. Spine Deform. 2022;10(1):31–44.
2. Li Z, Li X, Bi J, Chan MT, Wu WK, Shen J. Melatonin protected against the detrimental effects of microRNA-363 in a rat model of vitamin A-associated congenital spinal deformities: involvement of notch signaling. J Pineal Res. 2019;66(3):e12558.

3. Yang N, Wu N, Zhang L, Zhao Y, Liu J, Liang X, Ren X, Li W, Chen W, Dong S, Zhao S. TBX6 compound inheritance leads to congenital vertebral malformations in humans and mice. Hum Mol Genet. 2019;28(4):539–47.
4. Trapp B, de Andrade Lourenção Freddi T, de Oliveira Morais Hans M, Fonseca Teixeira Lemos Calixto I, Fujino E, Alves Rojas LC, Burlin S, Cerqueira Costa DM, Carrete Junior H, Abdala N, Tobaru Tibana LA. A practical approach to diagnosis of spinal dysraphism. Radiographics. 2021;41(2):559–75.
5. Cuny H, Rapadas M, Gereis J, Martin EM, Kirk RB, Shi H, Dunwoodie SL. NAD deficiency due to environmental factors or gene–environment interactions causes congenital malformations and miscarriage in mice. Proc Natl Acad Sci. 2020;117(7):3738–47.
6. Santiago FR, Ramos-Bossini AJ, Wáng YX, Zúñiga DL. The role of radiography in the study of spinal disorders. Quant Imaging Med Surg. 2020;10(12):2322–55.
7. Kim GU, Chang MC, Kim TU, Lee GW. Diagnostic modality in spine disease: a review. Asian Spine J. 2020;14(6):910–20.
8. Cuckle H, Maymon R. Development of prenatal screening—a historical overview. Semin Perinatol. 2016;40(1):12–22.
9. Brock D, Sutcliffe RG. Alpha-fetoprotein in the antenatal diagnosis of anencephaly and spina bifida. Lancet. 1972;300(7770):197–9.
10. Bernard JP, Cuckle HS, Stirnemann JJ, Salomon LJ, Ville Y. Screening for fetal spina bifida by ultrasound examination in the first trimester of pregnancy using fetal biparietaldiameter. Am J Obstet Gynecol. 2012;207(4):306–e1.
11. Bulas D. Fetal evaluation of spine dysraphism. Pediatr Radiol. 2010;40(6):1029–37.
12. Ghi T, Pilu G, Falco P, Segata M, Carletti A, Cocchi G, Santini D, Bonasoni P, Tani G, Rizzo N. Prenatal diagnosis of open and closed spinabifida. Ultrasound Obstet Gynecol. 2006;28(7):899–903.
13. Sepulveda W, Wong AE, Sepulveda F, Alcalde JL, Devoto JC, Otayza F. Prenatal diagnosis of spina bifida: from intracranial translucency to intrauterine surgery. Childs Nerv Syst. 2017;33(7):1083–99.
14. Sebire NJ, Noble PL, Thorpe-Beeston JG, Snijders RJ, Nicolaides KH. Presence of the 'lemon'sign in fetuses with spina bifida at the 10–14-week scan. Ultrasound Obstetr Gynecol. 1997;10(6):403–5.
15. Canick JA, Kellner LH, Bombard AT. Prenatal screening for open neural tube defects. Clin Lab Med. 2003;23(2):385–94.
16. Simon EM. MRI of the fetal spine. Pediatr Radiol. 2004;34(9):712–9.
17. Upasani VV, Ketwaroo PD, Estroff JA, Warf BC, Emans JB, Glotzbecker MP. Prenatal diagnosis and assessment of congenital spinal anomalies: review for prenatal counseling. World J Orthop. 2016;7(7):406–17.
18. Chao TT, Dashe JS, Adams RC, Keefover-Hicks A, McIntire DD, Twickler DM. Fetal spine findings on MRI and associated outcomes in children with open neural tube defects. Am J Roentgenol. 2011;197(5):W956–61.
19. Shekdar K, Feygin T. Fetal neuroimaging. Neuroimaging Clin. 2011;21(3):677–703.
20. Johnston LB, Borzyskowski M. Bladder dysfunction and neurological disability at presentation in closed spina bifida. Arch Dis Child. 1998;79(1):33–8.
21. Azzoni R, Gerevini S, Cabitza P. Spinal cord sonography in newborns: anatomy and diseases. J Pediatr Orthop B. 2005;14(3):185–8.
22. Babcook CJ. Ultrasound evaluation of prenatal and neonatal spina bifida. Neurosurg Clin N Am. 1995;6(2):203–18.
23. Pahys JM, Samdani AF, Betz RR. Intraspinal anomalies in infantile idiopathic scoliosis: prevalence and role of magnetic resonance imaging. Spine. 2009;34(12):E434–8.
24. Rajasekaran S, Kamath V, Kiran R, Shetty AP. Intraspinal anomalies in scoliosis: an MRI analysis of 177 consecutive scoliosis patients. Indian J Orthop. 2010;44(1):57–63.

25. Lowe LH, Johanek AJ, Moore CW. Sonography of the neonatal spine: part 1, Normal anatomy, imaging pitfalls, and variations that may simulate disorders. Am J Roentgenol. 2007;188(3):733–8.
26. Khanna JA, Wasserman BA, Sponseller PD. Magnetic resonance imaging of the pediatric spine. J Am Acad Orthop Surg. 2003;11(4):248–59.
27. Olsen EA, Brambrink AM. Anesthesia for the young child undergoing ambulatory procedures: current concerns regarding harm to the developing brain. Curr Opin Anesthesiol. 2013;26(6):677–84.
28. Reddy SV. Effect of general anesthetics on the developing brain. J Anaesthesiol Clin Pharmacol. 2012;28(1):6–10.
29. Antonov NK, Ruzal-Shapiro CB, Morel KD, Millar WS, Kashyap S, Lauren CT, Garzon MC. Feed and wrap MRI technique in infants. Clin Pediatr. 2017;56(12):1095–103.
30. Scrantin E, Robl T, Lindbichler F, Riccabona M. MRI of the neonatal and paediatric spine and spinal canal. Eur J Radiol. 2008;68(2):227–34.
31. Andronikou S, Wieselthaler N, Fieggen AG. Cervical spina bifida cystica: MRI differentiation of the subtypes in children. Childs Nerv Syst. 2006;22(4):379–84.

Chapter 4
Kyphosis

Ahmed Hassan A. Rady, Emry Atwa Ibrahim Mansour, Mohammedbaqer Ali Al-Ghuraibawi, and Ghazwan Abdulla Hasan

4.1 Introduction

Physiologically, kyphosis is the curvature of the angle between 20–40 °, so a curvature greater than 40 ° is considered pathologic kyphosis or hyper-kyphosis. A specific threshold between kyphosis and hyper-kyphosis is not established yet. The sagittal curvature of the spine is continuously altered throughout a person's life [1].

Conservative treatment is the first choice and if there are certain indications, surgical intervention is sought. Females have a higher incidence rate than males and it can occur in any age group, especially geriatrics. It could be due to variable factors such as traumatic, congenital malformation, disc degeneration, inflammation (inflammatory arthritis), infections, iatrogenic, or muscular, neuromuscular diseases. It is mainly due to the tension and compressive forces acting on the posterior and anterior aspects of the spine respectively and there are factors that resist these forces [2]. If

A. H. A. Rady (✉) · E. A. I. Mansour
Faculty of Medicine, Ain Shams University, El Weili, Egypt

M. A. Al-Ghuraibawi
Faculty of Medicine, University of Warith Al-Anbiyaa, Karbala, Iraq

G. A. Hasan
Royal Private Hospital, Baghdad, Iraq

K. F. AlAli, H. T. Hashim (eds.), *Congenital Spine Malformations*,
https://doi.org/10.1007/978-3-031-59031-3_4

any insult occurs to the anterior or posterior elements responsible for the normal curvature of the spine disrupting them, kyphosis will progress. It will occur because this disruption of the forces will lead to an increased rate of the lengthening of the posterior column relatively more than that of the anterior column. This will lead to the anterior movement of the center of gravity, as the spine's degree of curvature increases with its convexity posteriorly. When kyphosis becomes severe, the spinal cord may get tethered which is the most common cause of neurological manifestations. A detailed discussion will be conducted in this chapter about approaching patients with congenital kyphosis, Scheuermann kyphosis, post-laminectomy (post-surgical) kyphosis, kyphosis due to trauma, and Ankylosing spondylitis [3].

Cervical kyphosis: During embryological development, the human spine architecture gets its kyphotic shape. As a child learns to sit and hold hands upright, the secondary cervical and lumbar lordosis forms gradually. Normally the cervical lordosis is measured by the C2–C7 angle and falls between 10–20 °. Any deformity or significant deviations caused by any condition may lead to chronic pain, deformity of the spine, neurological diseases, and other complications may occur. To maintain a proper spine function, it is crucial to maintain a proper sagittal balance. A physiological vertebral body and intervertebral discs resist compression and bear about a third of the load, so any damage to the vertebral column for any cause as injury or degeneration may lead to kyphotic and lesser height column. The remaining two-thirds of the load is beared by the posterior elements to provide resistance to tension [4]. So any damage to these elements, posterior musculature, or ligamentous structures can lead to tension weakening and move stress to the anterior structures. Facets have an important role in maintaining this balance. As the spinal cord moves forward and stretches out over the posterior aspect of the vertebral body and intervertebral discs, this may lead to a compressed cord's vascular supply coupled with heightened tension within the cord, resulting in neuronal damage and myopathy may develop, which Is irreversible and fast-moving [5].

The iatrogenic cause is a common cause of kyphosis, mainly post-laminectomy kyphosis. This can occur due to any factor affecting the pathophysiological mechanism of kyphosis that we have discussed previously as insufficient restraints related to radiation therapy for tumors. Patients who have been diagnosed with post-laminectomy kyphosis report a temporary improvement [6]. This improvement is not long-lived and patients will have pain in the neck, forward head displacement, and severe neurological problems. A proper assessment of the patient is important to evaluate if there is any bowel or bladder dysfunction, as well as sexual dysfunction. In addition, it is necessary to assess a neurological examination to identify if there are any comparisons. A CT, plain radiography, and an MRI are useful to fully evaluate deformities. Not to forget that imaging study should be taken from many views, which are Anteroposterior, lateral, and flexion-extension views.

- MRI—useful to determine the spinal cord compression degree, disc degeneration, and collapse.
- CT—is useful for identifying bony ankylosis and vertebral artery anomalies.

While surgeons are planning for laminectomy, they should consider all various factors to minimize the risk possible for preventing post-operative kyphosis. Consider fusion in addition to decompression in patients with pre-operative instability, skeletal immaturity, multilevel decompression, and any amount of face resection.

In cases of patients without a neutral or lordotic spine on pre-operative lateral radiographs, they should not undergo posterior decompression as the spinal cord is unable to move away from the affected area. Kyphotic patients and in cases of neutral sagittal balance should undergo fusion along with decompression to restore anatomic alignment, which aids directly in a decompression. It is common to find kyphosis associated with other congenital conditions such as Larsen's syndrome, Klippel-Feil, myotonic dystrophy, osteogenesis imperfecta, and neurofibromatosis. Treatment protocol will differ according to the associated anomaly, it is crucial to be aware of them, if failure to identify anomalies may cause a grave prognosis [4].

Laren's syndrome: It is a rare congenital disorder characterized by short stature, abnormal facies, cleft lip and palate (full-thickness defect of lip or palate due to failure of facial prominence to fuse, cleft lip and palate usually occur together), and tracheomalacia. This syndrome may be associated with cervical kyphosis, anterior-posterior dissociations, and hypoplastic vertebrae. Surgical stabilization is required to prevent from progression of the deformity, recent researches suggest that non-operative treatment may be attempted early in life, although fusion will usually be necessary [7].

Klippel-Feil syndrome: Is characterized by a short, webbed neck, limited cervical spine range of motion, low hairline, Torticollis, facial asymmetry, and craniofacial abnormalities. Patients with this syndrome are usually present during childhood, diagnosis can be later in life. Kyphosis is not the only association with this syndrome, be aware that renal and cardiac anomalies also may be associated (common). Progressive kyphotic spine can lead to compression of the spinal cord and myelopathy as well, in these cases, evaluation by imaging study is a high benefit for pre-operative planning. The gold standard treatment for Klippel-Feil syndrome is surgery, as the non-operative treatment shows no beneficial or good outcomes [8].

4.2 Scheuermann's Kyphosis

Scheuermann's kyphosis represents a progressive kyphosis with more rigidity. It is not an uncommon cause of sagittal and angular progressive kyphosis, and mostly it affects children and adolescents. Scheuermann's kyphosis may present with back pain. Many theories have been suggested to explain the exact cause and mechanism of Scheuermann's kyphosis, unfortunately, the exact cause has not been understood yet, but it Is believed that it is due to a growth defectiveness of the end plate due to excessive mechanical stress during spinal growth. Many factors also may affect to development of Scheuermann's kyphosis. In the imaging study (radiographic features) we will observe anterior vertebral body wedging, irregularly shaped end plates, Schmorl's node (a bulge or protrusion of the vertebral disc jelly-like content into the growth cartilage of bone above and below the disc), and intervertebral disc degeneration. As the main or exact cause of Scheuermann's kyphosis is not well understood, the initial treatment is conservative management added to physiotherapy, rehabilitation, and bracing to prevent worsening the kyphotic deformity progression. If conservative treatment fails, surgery may be necessary [9].

4.3 Clinical Evaluation of Scheuermann's Kyphosis

Evaluation of approaching Scheuermann's kyphosis is a challenge as there are many confusing presentations of various classifications of kyphosis, so being aware of the characteristics of each type is crucial to reach spot diagnosis. For Scheuermann's type typically occurs during early adolescence, and because of the angular changes of the apex of the deformity, the kyphotic deformity associated with Scheuermann's disease remains visible when the spine is hyperextended. Other characteristics of these patients are that they present with small thoracolumbar scoliosis associated with primary thoracic kyphosis [10].

4.4 Clinical Presentation

- Pain that is intensified by standing or increased activity, the most severe pain is felt at the deformity's apex site, and commonly in the cervical and lumbar regions.
- Not associated with neurological deficits and comorbidities.
- Restrictive pulmonary disease due to the mechanical effects caused by larger deformities.

During the investigation by radiographic assessment, at least an anteroposterior (PA) view and lateral view should be taken. Normally, the sagittal measurements from the second thoracic vertebrae to the last thoracic vertebrae are from 10 ° to 40 °. On the other hand, the thoracolumbar region (T10–L2) is straight or slightly lordotic. Lumbar lordosis is between 50 and 70 ° and balances these thoracic and thoracolumbar measures in the sagittal plane. Typically, the plumb line from C7 should pass through the posterior superior corner of S1. Scheuermann's kyphosis involves thoracic and thoracolumbar curve patterns. The former is more rigid, with an apex at around T8 or T9. The latter is more discussed previously. This type of kyphosis should be differentiated from others such as degenerative flat back syndrome, as it is characterized mainly by multilevel degenerative disc disease rather than vertebral wedging. MRI also is highly important to identify any thoracic stenosis or disc herniation had been associated, that may affect the surgical plan [11].

Treatment of Scheuermann's kyphosis: Treatment could be operative or non-operative. Almost always the non-operative treatment is preferred. If Scheuermann's kyphosis presents no symptoms, no treatment is required, while kyphosis with greater than 75 or 80 ° requires a necessary treatment. Guidelines suggest a consideration of bracing if the curve is less than 75 ° in growing adolescents. Treatment should be accompanied by physiotherapy and exercises. Bracing should be worn for at least 18 h daily, and it should be taken off only while sleeping and necessaries.

Operation treatment: if non-operative treatment has no beneficial results, operation or surgical treatment may be necessary, especially for patients with advanced symptoms. Surgery aims to improve spinal balance, relieve pain, sagittal alignment improvement, higher the quality of life, and for cosmetic purposes [12].

4.5 Indications for Surgery

- Progressive deformity.
- Painful curve that progresses symptoms.
- Cosmetic purposes.
- Curve compresses and affects the cardiopulmonary functions.
- Neurological deficits.
- Curve with a degree greater than 75 °.

During the past decades, the surgical technique, and methods for treating Scheuermann's kyphosis have been improved significantly. Some techniques had shown limited achieving outcomes and maintained correction, as the Harrington compression and distraction instrumentation techniques, including Harrington non-segmental hook instrumentation, segmental hook instrumentation, sublaminar wires, and hybrid constructs using hook and screws were used for kyphosis correlation.

At various times, anterior and posterior techniques have shown favor, but current treatment is primarily using a posterior approach. The segmental bilateral pedicle screw fixation is the preferred technique for achieving kyphosis correlation. However, is performing adequate osseous-ligamentous releases, which are done using various osteotomy techniques. Posterior column osteotomies, in the form of smith-Peterson or Ponte osteotomies in the traumatic spine, and wide posterior releases, as described by Shufflebarger in the lumbar spine are the most useful and standard release techniques for Scheuermann's kyphosis disease. Also, the importance of the instrumentation allows more effective force application to the spine for deformity correction. The surgeon should evaluate the flexibility of the spine intraoperatively to determine whether more aggressive techniques are necessary as a pedicle subtraction osteotomy. Usually, the pedicle subtraction osteotomy is added in a condition that suffers from multilevel and stiff curves, or curves with a degree more than 100 °. When the surgeon completes the Ponte osteotomies, the lamina and then the pedicles bilaterally of the level requiring the pedicle subtraction osteotomy are excised. This is followed by the removal of a wedge-shaped piece of the vertebral body directly beneath the resected pedicles, resulting in an osseous release that will facilitate 30–40 ° of angular correction at the osteotomy site. One of the most crucial steps is selecting appropriate levels for instrumentation and fusion for the treatment of sagittal plane deformities. The second and third thoracic vertebrae are mainly chosen for upper instrumentation. The decision on the distal fusion level I is based on the sagittal sacral vertical plumb line that must bisect or nearly bisect the anticipated distal instrumented vertebra, this vertebra should be positioned distal to the first lordotic disc and rostral to a lordotic disc. Never forget to ensure that the first un-instrumentation too soon may result in distal junctional kyphosis (DJK), and it is may not be symptomatic, but it does always require revision surgery. Another issue with no clear etiology is the proximal junctional kyphosis. Generally, 50–60% correction of the deformity is adequate, as an over-correction may result in either proximal junctional kyphosis or DJK. The cervical and lumbar curves are expected to spontaneously correct themselves. It is important that (during Scheuermann's kyphosis correction surgery) the electro-physiologically spinal cord monitoring using all available techniques, including transcranial motor evoked potentials (TCMEP), somatosensory evoked potentials (SSEP), and pedicle screw stimulation. Additionally, optimizing vascular physiology during surgery is important to prevent deficits such as neurological deficits caused by disc herniation, osseous compressive pathologies, or vascular insults. Optimizing the hematocrit to ensure maximum oxygenation and increase the mean arterial pressure to 90 mmHg or higher, can achieve prevention. The neural canal must remain patent in cases where osteotomies are performed that may lead to large angular corrections, such as pedicle subtraction osteotomies or vertebral column resection [12].

Congenital kyphosis: An embryological disorder that represents either failure of formation of the vertebral body, failure of segmentation of the vertebral body, or formation failure with segmentation failure of the vertebral body (mixed between two malformations). Females have a greater incidence rate compared to males, and congenital kyphosis also with greater incidence rate compared with congenital scoliosis. The curvature apex is commonly between T10 and L1. The extent of kyphosis increases during the adolescent period, but the rate of progression decreases as soon as growth ceases. Failure of formation of the vertebral body leads to more apparent kyphosis than that caused by failure of segmentation. Chondrogenesis and ossification are the phases where congenital malformations of the vertebrae take place. If the growth rate of the epiphyseal endplate anterior to the transverse axis of the vertebrae is not adequate, congenital kyphosis occurs. Failure of formation of the vertebral body is the type which paraplegia is associated with the most which is due to the sharp angulation of the curvature of the spine. Paraplegia mostly occurs when the high rate of progression of kyphosis takes place during the adolescent period.

Post-laminectomy kyphosis: In cases of multiple cervical compressions or tumors, laminectomy involves lamina and part of vertebral bone that covers the spinal cord removal. This procedure has a side effect that may develop post-laminectomy kyphosis, especially following extensive laminectomy. The distribution of the load in the cervical region is not uniform (36% of the load to the forearm and 65% in the posterior column), so it is important to keep in mind that stability is disrupted when the posterior tension band is damaged. The posterior tension band involves the interspinous ligament, ligamentum flavum, and nuchal ligament. About 36% of children develop post-laminectomy kyphosis, which means that children are more likely to develop it than adults. Especially for children without facet damage. This percentage may be higher. Patients must be accurately selected for this procedure because this may be one of the main causes of post-laminectomy kyphosis [12, 13].

Many other factors may also reduce the risk of post-laminectomy kyphosis:

- Lordosis (10 ° or greater).
- Lack of instability found in the flexion and extension radiogram.
- Preservation of the facet during the surgery.

In conditions where the facets are unable to be protected, it is recommended to do a posterior fusion following decompression. Lateral mass screws represent the most common fusion methods. The rate of the instrumented posterior cervical fusion is more than 95%. Follow-up of the patients will highly reduce the risk of developing post-laminectomy kyphosis, accurate follow-up must be conducted.

Treatment: Three surgical strategies are used for managing post-laminectomy kyphosis:

- Anterior corpectomy and instrumentation.
- Posterior fusion and instrumentation.
- Combined anterior corpectomy and posterior fusion and instrumentation.

Conclusion: There is a high risk of progression to kyphosis after laminectomy is performed. This is because the different forces of the nuchal ligament, ligamentum flavum, and interspinous ligament (posterior tension band) that are responsible for stabilizing the spine are disrupted. Therefore, a high percentage of the children undergoing the laminectomy procedure develop kyphosis [14].

Post-traumatic kyphosis: Most commonly occurs in the thoracolumbar region. Occurs after a trauma of the spine or post-operatively. It may be due to the osteonecrosis of the vertebrae following the traumatic event which is known as Kümmel's disease [15–17]. The continuously developing neurological manifestations and pain indicate the need for a surgical operation. The surgical operation aims to return the anteroposterior curvature to the appropriate range and relieve the compressing forces acting on the nerves.

Ankylosing spondylitis: It is one of the chronic inflammatory rheumatic diseases that have systemic effects, these diseases including Ankylosing spondylitis, pseudoarthrosis, reactive arthritis, arthritis associated with inflammatory bowel disease, and undifferentiated spondyloarthropathies [18, 19]. The most common disease between them is Ankylosing spondylitis which affects the entire spine. Its prevalence ranges from 0.2% to 1.1%. Ankylosis spondylitis involves a major symptom represented by kyphosis, it involves the sacroiliac joint, the entire spine, major joints in the body, and extra-articular elements (enthesitis and uveitis). The most common affected area is the thoracic and lumbar region. Other symptoms of Ankylosing spondylitis are erosive disco vertebral lesions, and damage in the discs and vertebral bodies. The imaging study will show an erosion in the bone, sclerosis [20], syndesmophytes, ankylosis (bamboo spine), and osteoporosis.

Pain, joint stiffness, movement limitation, and respiratory distress, are other associated symptoms with Ankylosing spondylitis.

Non-operative treatment (medical therapy and exercise) can be useful to control the disease, while in a few cases, surgical treatment is necessary.

4.6 Indications for Surgical Treatment

- Unstable vertebral fractures.
- Myelopathy due to kyphotic progression.
- Progressive sagittal imbalance.

- Loss of horizontal gaze.
- Segmental instability.

Conclusion: Belongs to spondyloarthropathies which are systemic rheumatic diseases that cause chronic inflammation. The other four types are reactive arthritis, pseudoarthrosis, undifferentiated spondyloarthropathies, and arthritis associated with inflammatory bowel disease. Thoracic and lumbar parts of the spine are affected the most although Ankylosing Spondylitis commonly affects the whole spine. The vertebrae and the intervertebral discs are eroded by these diseases which eventually lead to kyphosis. Pain throughout the spine is the most common symptom experienced.

4.7 Clinical Presentation/Complications

- Extreme curvature of the spine with posterior convexity.
- Deteriorated physical ability.
- Limited range of motion.
- Pain due to altered sagittal plane.
- Poor quality of life.
- Pulmonary compromise.
- Breathing difficulty.

4.8 Diagnostic Investigations

To diagnose Kyphosis a physical exam is performed with known clinical representations as stated above this may be followed by an X-ray imaging. From a diagnostic point of view, Kyphosis is defined as a curvature of the spine measuring 50 ° or greater on an X-ray image. The normal spine usually bends from 20 ° to 45 ° of curvature in the upper back area.

4.9 Examination

Physical Exam: During the physical exam, the doctor looks at your back and palpates the spine for any abnormalities or muscle tenderness. Tenderness is seen by pressing on the muscles, but t best notice or view kyphosis an Adam's Forward Bending Test performed where the patient is asked to bend forward from the waist and the back is observed from the side, and other neurological tests can be done to test for any neural defects (Checking patient's reflexes and muscle strength) [21, 22].

4.10 Imaging

X-rays or CT scans can be ordered for the patients to view the degree of curvature of the spine hence the severity of the condition and to check for any abnormalities in the vertebrate. Usually, an X-ray is enough but a CT-Scan can be ordered for a better view with more details. For the etiology MRI imaging can be used to detect infection or a tumor in the spine [23, 24].

4.11 Other Tests

Bone Density test: Low-density bone can worsen kyphosis and often can be improved with medications.

Nerve test (INCASE IN NERVE AFFECTION).

4.12 Treatment

Kyphosis treatment depends on the cause and severity of the patient's condition. Most kyphosis cases don't require any treatments [24, 25].

4.13 Physical Therapy and Exercise

Some types of kyphosis can be improved with the use of physical therapy that includes Stretching, strengthening exercises, and posture training that works on improving spinal flexibility and relieving pain. In other kyphosis cases, the etiology must be treated but Physical therapy is important to prevent worsening kyphosis due to the progressive nature of kyphosis with aging [26]. In children with a case of Scheuermann's disease wearing a spine brace will be able to stop the progression of kyphosis while their bones are still growing [27].

4.14 Medications

As mentioned above the treatment of kyphosis mainly depends on the cause and severity of the condition. But kyphosis treatment may include OTC pain-relieving drugs such as acetaminophen (Tylenol, others), ibuprofen (Advil, Motrin IB, others), or naproxen sodium (Aleve), in case of ineffectiveness stronger substitutes will be given by prescription. Also, Osteoporotic drugs are prescribed to strengthen patients' bones to avoid spinal fractures that may worsen the condition [28].

4.15 Surgery

In severe cases where kyphosis has affected the nervous system (spinal cord or nerve roots), surgery is required with Spinal Fusion Surgeries being the most common [29–31].

Multiple Choice Questions

1. **A two-year-old male presented with painful and rigid kyphotic deformity of the cervical region for an onset of 3 weeks, associated with bowel and bladder issues. What is the most appropriate investigation you would send the patient for:**

   A. Angiograph.
   B. Magnetic resonance imaging.
   C. X-ray.
   D. Blood test to look for infection.
   E. Pulmonary function test to ensure kyphosis is compressing on the chest.

2. **A patient came to you as a surgeon for a consultation to do surgery, the patient suffers from joint stiffness, movement limitation, respiratory distress, and pain in the major body joints including the hip joint and shoulders. He was diagnosed by his doctor with Ankylosing spondylitis. According to this case, all the following are indications for a surgical treatment Except:**

   A. Progressive sagittal imbalance.
   B. Myelopathy due to kyphotic progression.
   C. Succeed non-operative therapy.
   D. Segmental instability.
   E. Unstable vertebral fractures.

3. **A twenty-year-old male came to the clinic suffering from lower back pain, and lower limb numbness, with no surgical history or trauma. He was diagnosed with Scheuermann's kyphosis. According to his case, which of the following is not correct about surgical indications:**

   A. Curve with a degree greater than 75 °.
   B. Curve compresses and affects the cardiopulmonary functions.
   C. Progressive deformity.
   D. The patient needs cosmetic correlation.
   E. Curve with a degree greater than 25 °.

4. **According to congenital kyphosis, which of the following statements is not correct:**

   A. An embryological disorder represents either failure of formation of the vertebral body, failure of segmentation of the vertebral body, or formation failure with segmentation failure of the vertebral body (mixed between two malformations).

B. The extent of kyphosis increases during the adolescent period.
C. The curvature apex is commonly between T10 and L1.
D. Males have a higher incidence rate than females.
E. Chondrogenesis and ossification are the phases where congenital malformations of the vertebrae take place.

5. **A patient came to the clinic with a suspected kyphosis symptom, according to his case, which of the following is not a specific symptom for kyphosis:**

A. Breathing difficulty.
B. Leg ulcer.
C. Limited range of motion.
D. Extreme curvature of the spine with posterior convexity.
E. Deteriorated physical ability.

6. **A female child who has short stature, abnormal facies, cleft lip and palate, and tracheomalacia. She was diagnosed with cervical kyphosis. According to her associated symptoms, she mostly has:**

A. Marfan's syndrome.
B. Down syndrome.
C. Laren's syndrome.
D. Klippel-Feil syndrome.
E. Vitamin B12 deficiency.

7. **A kyphotic female patient suffering from a short, webbed neck, limited cervical spine range of motion, low hairline, Torticollis, facial asymmetry, and craniofacial abnormalities. According to her symptoms, her condition is mostly associated with:**

A. Laren's syndrome.
B. Klippel-Feil syndrome.
C. Vitamin B12 deficiency.
D. Endocrine issue.
E. Hypothyroidism.

8. **Laminectomy is a surgery with a great risk of developing post-laminectomy kyphosis, so selecting a patient to have this surgery must be done accurately, if you are a surgeon, what are the cases that you will accept this procedure:**

A. Central canal stenosis.
B. Laminectomy with lateral recess decompression and foraminotomy to completely decompress the lateral recess.
C. When symptoms derived from stenosis do not respond to conservative treatment.
D. For cosmetic purposes.
E. Primary or secondary tumors.

9. **According to the imaging study that we use to diagnose kyphosis, all the following statements are not correct except:**
   A. MRI is useful to determine the spinal cord compression degree, disc degeneration, and collapse.
   B. CT is useful to determine the spinal cord compression degree, disc degeneration, and collapse.
   C. X-ray is required to determine the spinal cord compression degree, disc degeneration, and collapse.
   D. An angiogram is the first investigation's best choice.
   E. It is enough to take an image from only one view.

10. **Regarding kyphosis, all the following statements are correct except:**
    A. Females are more affected than males.
    B. When evaluating an imaging study, it is preferred to evaluate it from more than one view.
    C. Kyphosis may cause compression in the chest which can lead to breathing difficulties.
    D. Hyper-kyphosis is defined as a curve of 30 ° or less.
    E. Ankylosing spondylitis is one of the chronic inflammatory rheumatic diseases that have systemic effects.

References

1. Bettany-Saltikov J, de Mauroy JC. Kyphosis physiotherapy from childhood to old age. In: Physical therapy perspectives in the 21st century—challenges and possibilities. INTECH Open Access Publisher; 2012.
2. Fon GT, Pitt MJ, Thies AC. Thoracic kyphosis: range in normal subjects. Am J Roentgenol. 1980;134(5):979–83. https://doi.org/10.2214/ajr.134.5.979.
3. Katzman WB, Wanek L, Shepherd JA, Sellmeyer DE. Age-related hyperkyphosis: its causes, consequences, and management. J Orthop Sports Phys Ther. 2010;40(6):352–60. https://doi.org/10.2519/jospt.2010.3099.
4. Koelé MC, Lems WF, Willems HC. The clinical relevance of hyperkyphosis: a narrative review. Front Endocrinol. 2020;11 https://doi.org/10.3389/fendo.2020.00005.
5. Yaman O, Dalbayrak S. Kyphosis and review of the literature. Turk Neurosurg. 2013; https://doi.org/10.5137/1019-5149.jtn.8940-13.0.
6. Heary RF, Albert TJ. Spinal deformities: the essentials. Thieme; 2014.
7. Marks DS, Qaimkhani SA. The natural history of congenital scoliosis and kyphosis. Spine. 2009;34(17):1751–5. https://doi.org/10.1097/brs.0b013e3181af1caf.
8. Kirollos R, Helmy A, Thomson S, Hutchinson PJA. Oxford textbook of neurological surgery. Oxford University Press; 2019.
9. Van Goethem JWM, van den Hauwe L, Parizel PM. Spinal imaging: diagnostic imaging of the spine and spinal cord. Springer; 2010.
10. Culham EG, Jimenez HA, King CE. Thoracic kyphosis, Rib mobility, and lung volumes in normal women and women with osteoporosis. Spine. 1994;19(11):1250–5. https://doi.org/10.1097/00007632-199405310-00010.

11. Edmondston SJ, Singer KP. Thoracic spine: anatomical and biomechanical considerations for manual therapy. Man Ther. 1997;2(3):132–43. https://doi.org/10.1054/math.1997.0293.
12. Albert TJ, Vacarro A. Postlaminectomy kyphosis. Spine. 1998;23:2738–45.
13. Bell GR, Stearns KL. Flexion-extension MRI of the upper rheumatoid cervical spine. Orthopedics. 1991;14:969–73; discussion 973–974
14. Boden SD, Dodge LD, Bohlman HH, Rechtine GR. Rheumatoid arthritis of the cervical spine. A long-term analysis with predictors of paralysis and recovery. J Bone Joint Surg Am. 1993;75:1282–97.
15. Chamberlain W. Basilar impression (platybasia). A bizarre developmental anomaly of the occipital bone and upper cervical spine with striking and misleading neurologic manifestations. Yale J Biol Med. 1939;11:487–96.
16. Clark CR, Goetz DD, Menezes AH. Arthrodesis of the cervical spine in rheumatoid arthritis. J Bone Joint Surg Am. 1989;71:381–92.
17. Currier BL. Surgical management of cervical spine instability. Curr Opin Rheumatol. 1990;2:176–87.
18. Hilibrand AS, Tannenbaum DA, Graziano GP, Loder RT, Hensinger RN. The sagittal alignment of the cervical spine in adolescent idiopathic scoliosis. J Pediatr Orthop. 1995;15:627–32.
19. Katsumi Y, Honma T, Nakamura T. Analysis of cervical instability resulting from laminectomies for removal of spinal cord tumor. Spine. 1989;14:1171–6.
20. Lonstein JE. Post-laminectomy kyphosis. Clin Orthop Relat Res. 1977;128:93–100.
21. McRae DL, Barnum AS. Occipitalization of the atlas. Am J Roentgenol Radium Therapy Nucl Med. 1953;70:23–46.
22. Panjabi MM. The stabilizing system of the spine. Part I. Function, dysfunction, adaptation, and enhancement. J Spinal Disord. 1992;5:383–9; discussion 397
23. Panjabi MM. The stabilizing system of the spine. Part II. Neutral zone and instability hypothesis. J Spinal Disord. 1992;5:390–6; discussion 397
24. Panjabi MM, Thibodeau LL, Crisco JJ III, White AA III. What constitutes spinal instability? Clin Neurosurg. 1988;34:313–39.
25. Ranawat CS, O'Leary P, Pellicci P, Tsairis P, Marchisello P, Dorr L. Cervical spine fusion in rheumatoid arthritis. J Bone Joint Surg Am. 1979;61:1003–10.
26. McGregor M. The significance of certain measurements of the skull in the diagnosis of basilar impression. Br J Radiol. 1948;21:171–81.
27. Redlund-Johnell I, Pettersson H. Radiographic measurements of the cranio-vertebral region. Designed for evaluation of abnormalities in rheumatoid arthritis. Acta Radiol Diagn. 1984;25:23–8.
28. Riew KD, Hilibrand AS, Palumbo MA, Sethi N, Bohlman HH. Diagnosing basilar invagination in the rheumatoid patient. The reliability of radiographic criteria. J Bone Joint Surg Am. 2001;83-A:194–200.
29. Zdeblick TA, Abitbol JJ, Kunz DN, McCabe RP, Garfin S. Cervical stability after sequential capsule resection. Spine. 1993;18:2005–8.
30. Zdeblick TA, Zou D, Warden KE, McCabe R, Kunz D, Vanderby R. Cervical stability after foraminotomy. Abiomechanical in vitro analysis. J Bone Joint Surg Am. 1992;74:22–7.
31. Riew KD, Hilibrand AS, Palumbo MA, Bohlman HH. Anterior cervical corpectomy in patients previously managed with a lamina tomy: short-term complications. J Bone Joint Surg Am. 1999;81(7):950–7.

Chapter 5
Lordosis

Mohamad Abdulwahab Sabsabee and Ahmed Ameer Mohammed

Test your learning and check your understanding of this book's contents: use the "Springer Nature Flashcards" app to access questions using ▶ https://sn.pub/QCsfpd.
To use the app, please follow the instructions in Chap. 1.

5.1 Introduction

Congenital spinal malformations remain a challenge to orthopedic surgeons as research and literature regarding this topic are yet to be fulfilled. Among different spinal deformities, congenital lordosis is the least appreciated although it has a high mortality rate, if not the highest, thus, early detection and treatment are of vital importance [1].

It is defined as an abnormal spinal column development in the sagittal plane that is present since birth, thus, a noticeable curvature might be seen earlier in the life of the affected children. With that being said, early and timely diagnosis is important before the development of a severe curve.

5.2 Mechanism

It usually happens as a result of the failure of segmentation of the posterior compartment involving multiple levels of vertebrae combined with anterior plates' active growth. This leads to the fusion of the posterior laminar and articular parts and the

M. A. Sabsabee (✉) · A. A. Mohammed
Sulaiman Alrajhi University, Al Bukayriyah, Saudi Arabia

K. F. AlAli, H. T. Hashim (eds.), *Congenital Spine Malformations*,
https://doi.org/10.1007/978-3-031-59031-3_5

formation of an unsegmented bar. If the unsegmented bar is posterolateral, the resulting deformity is lordoscoliosis. Another proposed mechanism is the formation failure of the posterior segment; however, this mechanism is extremely rare with some authors stating that they didn't see a single case. This increase in anterior plates growth alters the distance between the spine and the sternum resulting in decreased space and modification of the mechanics involved in the movement of the thoracic cage. This ultimately leads to restriction of pulmonary function, respiratory failure, core pulmonale, and if not recognized early death [2].

5.3 Epidemiology

The accepted prevalence of congenital spinal malformations in the literature is approximately 0.5–1 in 1000 live births, which is considered rare. There are no reported statistics regarding congenital lordosis as a separate entity. Information available states that it is the least common presentation identified. Moreover, pure lordosis due to failure of segmentation is rare and the same deformity as a result of the failure of formation is even extremely rare. On the other hand, Posterolateral failure of segmentation resulting in lordoscoliosis is more commonly encountered [1–3].

5.4 Etiology

Why this congenital deformity happens is usually not clear and is thought to take place due to multiple reasons. One of these reasons is intrauterine abnormalities caused by maternal exposure to diabetes, alcohol, carbon monoxide, anti-epileptic medications, and infection. Another proposed cause is errors in genetics and morphogenesis. However, the deformity will usually be identified as part of an associated syndrome like Goldenhar, Jarcho-Levin, Klippel-Feil, and VACTERL (vertebral, anal atresia, cardiac, tracheoesophageal fistula, renal, and limb anomalies) [4].

5.5 Patient's Presentation

Patients presenting with pure congenital lordosis have an insidious presentation. The deformity is usually severe and the curve is progressive with a greater effect on pulmonary function, especially in thoracic lordosis. A compromised pulmonary function can be in the picture of an increased work of breathing, inability to breathe while lying prone, decreased lung compliance, decreased vital capacity, increased pulmonary arterial pressure, and mismatched ventilation-perfusion ratio. In patients with lordoscoliosis, the effect on pulmonary function is directly related to the degree of the lordosis measured. Winter et al. reported five cases of lordoscoliosis with significant thoracic lordosis and compromised pulmonary function. He noticed an improvement in the vital capacity of those whose surgical treatment was directed at correcting the thoracic lordosis. On the other hand, those who got surgical treatment directed at correcting the lateral curvature did not show any improvement in their pulmonary function. The bottom line is that pulmonary function is directly related to the degree of lordosis and the anteroposterior diameter of the chest. A patient can also present with an associated isolated congenital anomaly or syndrome which are described above [3–6].

5.6 Work up

Evaluation of patients with congenital spinal deformity should start with careful and complete history followed by a thorough physical examination. The aim is to define the pathology and to look for any associated anomalies. It is also important to know if the curve is progressive or not, and the rate of that progression. The spinal growth rate is highest in the first 3 years of life and during the adolescent growth spurt and is directly linked to the rate of progression of the curve, so greater care should be taken when the patient presents during those periods. Since patients are usually young, birth history and developmental milestones are of great importance. Weight should be recorded alongside the sitting and standing height. The complete balance of the spine should be assessed in both the sagittal and coronal plane clinically and with the aid of imaging techniques. This includes head tilt, shoulder symmetry, sitting balance, and pelvic balance. The rigidity of the curve should also be assessed clinically with careful inspection of the thoracic cage to look for any asymmetry [1, 3, 4].

Associated anomalies should be kept in mind when evaluating the patient. It is recommended to perform an ultrasound of the genitourinary tract to look for any anomalies as well as an echocardiogram with full clinical cardiac evaluation to identify any cardiac pathologies.

Last but not least, a pulmonary function test should be obtained in all patients who are presenting with restricted pulmonary function, especially thoracic lordosis patients. If the patient can't tolerate a pulmonary function test, CT lung volumes and dynamic MRI would be required [5].

5.7 Complications

Since congenital lordosis patients have usually an affected pulmonary function, the resulting complication is usually a respiratory failure, COR pulmonale, and early death. In case surgical intervention was performed, increased blood loss, arrhythmias, and superficial infection have been reported [6, 7].

5.8 Associated Conditions

Congenital spinal deformities (including congenital lordosis) are associated with many conditions. Some of them are benign while others are life-threatening. Intraspinal anomalies can accompany congenital lordosis in up to 35% of cases. Some examples of these anomalies are stenosis, diastematomyelia, and spinal cord tethering which could limit surgical intervention. Signs that could suggest presence of intraspinal anomaly include asymmetrical limb deformities, neurological deficits, and posterior skin lesions. Isolated Congenital Defects can also accompany congenital spinal deformity. They could affect the cardiovascular, renal, musculoskeletal, gastrointestinal systems. A detailed history coupled with a through physical examination can reveal most of them. Additional testing and imaging may be required to fully exclude some defects. Echocardiography, renal ultrasound, and brain and spine MRI are essential for most cases. Although the genetic component is not yet fully understood, some syndromes found to be associated with spinal deformity; VATER, Goldenhar, Poland's, Noonan, CHARGE are some examples. In addition, congenital lordosis could the manifestation of a connective tissue disease such as Larsen syndrome. The take away point is to treat the patient in a holistic approach. All of these conditions must be identified and treated accordingly; as a lot can, be more concerning for the patient's wellbeing or affect the treatment plan [1, 5, 8].

5.9 Treatment

Mostly, lordosis is accompanied with another primary defect and treatment should tailored to the primary defect. Rarely, when lordosis present as the primary defect only viable option is surgery. Conservative treatment does not play any role in the treatment of this progressive deformity. Emphasis should be placed on early intervention to prevent serious deformity and complications. All patients require anterior approach as anterior growth is the main mechanism of deformation. However, this anterior approach carries a greater risk because almost all of these patients have restrictive lung disease. In addition to that, surgery is contraindicated in those who suffer from pulmonary artery hypertension (PAH) because of the high mortality rate. There are two types of procedures which can be done. Anterior fusion which can halt the progression of lordosis. The other one is corrective adopting both anterior and posterior approaches [1, 3, 7, 8].

5.9.1 Anterior Fusion

This approach is used when the deformity presents early before the development of significant pulmonary impairment to prevent further progression. Stunting growth is not a concern here because it is already being affected by the deformity itself. The anterior fusion procedure includes: vertebral discs excision followed by cartilage endplates removal then using bone chips to pack the emptied disc spaces. This anterior fusion process should be applied to the whole affected area and one or two vertebrae superiorly and inferiorly. This process will result in elimination of any further anterior growth and ensure fusion opposite to the unsegmented bar [7].

5.9.2 Corrective Surgery

Corrective approach is the choice for those with significant deformity and, deteriorating lung function. It aims to restore spinal alignment and improve the pulmonary function by combining anterior and posterior approaches. When possible, the two approach should be combined under the same anesthetic session to maximize the immediate improvement in pulmonary function. It differs from the aforementioned anterior fusion procedure. Anteriorly, excision of all discs in the affected area is done. After that, it will be converted into an osteotomy by excising thin wedges of the adjacent vertebral endplates. The difference is no bone chips packing is required as the wedges have to close anteriorly. Posteriorly, the procedure includes multiple osteotomies of the laminar synostosis. These have to match the anteriorly excised discs levels. The next step is to pass sublaminar wires which can guide the spine into a kyphotically contoured rod. The goal is to achieve a balanced spine alongside a stable thoracic cage. Advantages include allowing growth by delaying spinal fusion. Moreover, spinal mobility is preserved by decreasing the number of vertebral segments included in the fusion [8].

5.10 Prognosis

This condition is progressive, and if left untreated can lead to catastrophic outcomes. As it progresses, it will affect the lung capacity and function leading ultimately to death. If discovered and treated early, patients can have good quality of life [1, 5, 8].

Multiple Choice Questions

1. **What is the most common mechanism of congenital lordosis?**

    A. Failure of formation
    B. Mixed mechanism
    C. Unsegmented bar
    D. Block vertebra

    Answer: C

2. **When looking at pure congenital lordosis, how common is it?**

   A. Very common
   B. Uncommon
   C. Rare
   D. Extremely rare

   Answer: C

3. **All choices are associated anomalies with congenital lordosis except?**

   A. Genito urological anomaly
   B. Cardiac anomaly
   C. Intraspinal anomaly
   D. Hepatic anomaly

   Answer: D

4. **Spinal growth rate is increased in adolescence and in….?**

   A. The first 3 years of life
   B. After entering primary school
   C. After 25 years of age
   D. After 40 years of age

   Answer: A

5. **What is the best modality for a detailed description of the spinal column deformity?**

   A. Lateral radiograph
   B. 3D CT scan
   C. Posteroanterior standing radiograph
   D. MRI

   Answer: B

6. **What is the optimal conservative line of management for congenital lordosis?**

   A. Physiotherapy
   B. Watchful waiting
   C. Bracing
   D. No role for conservative management

   Answer: D

7. **What is the best surgical approach for early detected cases?**

   A. Anterior fusion
   B. Posterior fusion
   C. Combined approach
   D. Hemivertebra excision

   Answer: A

8. **What is the best surgical approach for advanced cases?**

   A. Anterior fusion
   B. Posterior fusion
   C. Combined approach
   D. Hemivertebra excision

   Answer: C

9. **What is the deforming mechanism of congenital lordosis?**

   A. Anterior growth
   B. Posterior growth
   C. Axial load
   D. Muscle weakness

   Answer: A

10. **Which of these investigations should done for all congenital lordosis patients at time of initial diagnosis?**

    A. ECG
    B. CBC
    C. Abdomen CT
    D. Abdominal US

    Answer: D

References

1. Basu PS, Elsebaie H, Noordeen M. Congenital spinal deformity. Spine. 2002;20:2255–9. https://doi.org/10.1097/00007632-200210150-00014.
2. Loughenbury PR, Gummerson NW, Tsirikos AI. Congenital spinal deformity: assessment, natural history and treatment. Orthop Trauma. 2017;6:364–9. https://doi.org/10.1016/j.mporth.2017.09.007.
3. Chan G, Dormans JP. Update on congenital spinal deformities. Spine. 2009;17:1766–74. https://doi.org/10.1097/BRS.0b013e3181ab62d8.
4. Winter RB, Moe JH, Bradford DS. Congenital thoracic lordosis. J Bone Joint Surg. 1978;6:806–10. https://doi.org/10.2106/00004623-197860060-00014.
5. Winter RB, Leonard AS. Surgical correction of congenital thoracic lordosis. J Pediatr Orthop. 1990;6:805–8. https://doi.org/10.1097/01241398-199011000-00020.
6. Giampietro PF, Raggio CL, Blank RD, McCarty C, Broeckel U, Pickart MA. Clinical, genetic and environmental factors associated with congenital vertebral malformations. Mol Syndromol. 2012;4(1–2):94–105. https://doi.org/10.1159/000345329.
7. Kanagaraju V, Chhabra HS, Srivastava A, Mahajan R, Kaul R, Bhatia P, et al. A case of severe and rigid congenital thoracolumbar lordoscoliosis with diastematomyelia presenting with type 2 respiratory failure: managed by staged correction with controlled axial traction. Eur Spine J. 2014;25(10):3034–41. https://doi.org/10.1007/s00586-014-3624-0.
8. Lonstein JE. Congenital spine deformities. Orthop Clin N Am. 1999;30(3):387–405. https://doi.org/10.1016/s0030-5898(05)70094-8.

Chapter 6
Scoliosis

Vanya Ibrahim Jwamer, Kani Ahmed, Ghazwan Abdulla Hasan, and Ahmed Dheyaa Al-Obaidi

Test your learning and check your understanding of this book's contents: use the "Springer Nature Flashcards" app to access questions using ▶ https://sn.pub/QCsfpd.
To use the app, please follow the instructions in Chap. 1.

6.1 Introduction

Adult scoliosis defined as deformity or deviation in the skeletal spine of mature patient, normally human beings have curves like cervical and lumber lordosis with thoracic kyphosis, in scoliosis spinal curvature with cobb angle more than 10 ° [1, 2] if less than 10 ° it's called asymmetry in the spine [2], and this abnormality associated with thoracolumbar curvature as compensatory, and most of time its associated with lordosis or kyphosis [3, 4].

The exact cause is unknown, and we have some types of the scoliosis:

Congenital scoliosis, idiopathic scoliosis, degenerative scoliosis.

Congenital scoliosis: Is a developmental abnormality related to spine either failure of formation or segmentation or both, and malformation of the other systems

V. I. Jwamer (✉) · K. Ahmed
School of Medicine, University of Sulaimani, Sulaymaniyah, Iraq

G. A. Hasan
Royal Private Hospital, Baghdad, Iraq

A. D. Al-Obaidi
College of Medicine, University of Baghdad, Baghdad, Iraq

K. F. AlAli, H. T. Hashim (eds.), *Congenital Spine Malformations*,
https://doi.org/10.1007/978-3-031-59031-3_6

often seen, and we can diagnose them by MRI and the treatment is follow up or surgery before development of the large curve [5, 6].

Idiopathic scoliosis: Affects nearly 2% of the patients, its more in the adult patient and the cause is unknown, the curvature in this type is >500, so history and examination is very important with the modalities of the diagnosis and treatment to decide for surgical correction or not and better outcome and less complication for the patient [7–9].

Neuromuscular scoliosis: Is common condition in those disease that cause muscle hypotonia and contracture like spinal muscular dystrophy and Cerebral palsy, Duchene muscular dystrophy, this type of scoliosis is difficult with more complication, and our aim is to prevent it with physiotherapy and preventing the contracture, for the treatment mainly its surgery with better outcome [10], the deformed spine with this disease lead to impairment in the other systems as well as daily live activity and according to the part that affecting by the abnormality [11].

Degenerative scoliosis: This type more common in the old age female patient, its multifactorial illness, degeneration of the disc and the facets leads to asymmetric degeneration and symptoms, when the cobb angle is >30° so its curve progression [12, 13].

6.2 Clinical Presentation

Back pain: the most common symptoms in scoliosis and its unclear [14], mostly its due to spinal canal stenosis because there may be disc herniation or hypertrophy of the ligaments and osteophyte that pressing the canal and leads to stenosis and pain [9].

Claudication: mainly this symptom due to stenosis of the canal that pressing the nerve and causing claudication which's worse during standing and relive during sitting and bending forward if its severe so affect the bladder control mechanism and cauda equina syndrome, this claudication is neuronal so we should differentiate it from the vascular one, the vascular commonly associated with vascular disease and absent distant pulse [15, 16].

Radicular symptoms: this symptom mainly due to spinal stenosis also, the osteophyte formation, disc herniation, and ligament hypertrophy leads to this stenosis and radical pain and stretching of the nerve [14].

Disabilities: these symptoms produce due to excess muscle strain because these patients will need greater effort to stand up and move, when the curvature is more its associated with cardiopulmonary problems especially when cobb angle >500 [17].

6.3 History and Examination

History is important part for scoliosis with the patients presentation and we should take it in the chronological manner, asking about onset site, duration, intensity, radiation, aggravating and reliving factor, and age of the patient because degenerative type is more in the old age while the idiopathic type is more in the younger age groups, and other systems function like bowel, bladder, change in memory, motor function and sensory function [18] about previous surgery, the type, and complication of the surgery or the hospital stay, also asking about cardiopulmonary or vascular problems, and the gait of the patients with the shape of back and shoulder in standing position, the normal curvature should be inspected like lumber lordosis an thoracic kyphosis, limb length discrepancy, palpation of the bony pelvis and checking pain.

For the examinations we start from the general examination then we proceed to the specific examinations, neurological exam, vital sign, cardiopulmonary exams we ask the patient to stand and checking for balance, for the coronal balance we inspect shoulders of the patient while for the sagittal balance we inspect the normal curvatures, and palpation for pain detection and muscle tenderness with spasm, we should see the patient while changing positions and during flat lying and leg extension, with examinations of the joints, examining the myotomes and dermatome, vascular examination and in prone position we prefer examination for surgery assessment [19, 20].

6.4 Modalities of Diagnosis of Scoliosis

6.4.1 Diagnosis Depends on Clinical Evaluation and Imaging Techniques

Radiographic evaluation is the fundamental component in diagnosing, monitoring the changes that occur with growth and managing lumber scoliosis. Although plain conventional radiographs are usually adequate in the initial evaluation of spine deformity, the surgeons nowadays are equipped with several other tools to assess a patient radiographically with clinical correlation based on history and physical examination, the new tools that are advanced imaging modalities include computed tomography (CT scan) and magnetic resonance imaging (MRI).

6.4.2 X-Ray

Plain radiographs are crucial in the evaluation of bony morphology, commonly this modality may be the only imaging required for the assessment of lumber scoliosis specifically in patients with no history of spine surgery and the deformity limited to lumber spine.

Plain film radiography is the major appliance in diagnosing spinal deformity particularly in adults with lumber scoliosis. In the community and at first presentation plain X-rays are the essential modality for the assessment after history and physical examinations it's cheap and available.

The basic evaluation includes global and regional assessment with AP and lateral views from C2 to pelvis including femoral heads; typically, full-body imaging is taken in upright, unsupported, weight-bearing position, this will show the true degree of deformity in axial loading [21–23], activation of compensatory mechanisms, and other pathology which may be part of the reason of the pain and disability [24].

The ultimate advantage of X-ray is the ability to calculate the angle of torsion using the Cobb method and monitoring morphological advances in the vertebrae [25]. Cobb Method is the process of selecting the most affected vertebrae (with the most rotation) which is the bone having biggest diversion from a straight line in the curve with the least amount of tilt calling it the Apical Vertebrae, also locating the vertebrae with the most tilt above and below the apical vertebrae of the curve and drawing a line at top edge of the above vertebrae and lower edge of the below vertebrae both extending out at the angle of the vertebrae [26, 27]. The cobb angle is needed for measuring the initial curve follow up and the need for surgery, an angle of at least 10 is required for diagnosis [28] Cobb angle can be affected by radiologist's experience [29] and has a measurement error of up to 11.8 ° [30].

One of the simpler diagnostic procedures is the Adams forward bend test that assesses posture and identifies scoliosis, which is part of functional tests its short, non-invasive painless and doesn't need instruments used by medical personnel, the patient is required to bend down and the medical personnel standing behind the patient looks at the back of the patient across the spine's horizontal plane, this test can recognize scoliosis in its advanced stages and not very beneficial in its earlier stages [31] X-ray's radiation has damaging effects which will prolong the course of diagnosis over time [32]. Nowadays the dose of radiation is less but the number of x rays taken at the time of diagnosis or during adolescence in children is at least 12 times, which will have accumulated effect leading to higher cancer rates in children than adults [33–35]. And doctors are not able to follow up the treatment process accurately or whether the results are as needed [36].

That's why the optimal diagnosing method is computer diagnostic tools since they are detailed and non-invasive without the adverse effects of radiation [37] computerized approaches are of reasonable abundance since they are able to detect scoliosis even in its early stages with the first signs of curvature and pinpoint the problem by allowing all planes of the body to be inspected [38, 39].

6.4.3 CT Scan

X—rays use 2D images but the progress in medicine and technology have led to the advancement of new essential 3D techniques using CT or MRI [40, 41]. CT like X-ray is a procedure that uses radiation to produce cross sectional images but has better assessment of bony and soft tissue structures which is at a price of higher radiation liability [42]. Despite the disadvantages of CT it provides excellent axial imaging showing Rotational deformity [43]. Decisions for operation are largely guided by CT imaging because it provides detailed evaluation for Apical rotation degree which is prognostic for progress [44, 45] and affects rigidity of the curve [46], Because of the high radiation and to prevent over exposure to radiation the cross sections are taken at the level of the border of vertebrae, vertebral column and pelvis [47], CT compared to MRI is faster, lower cost, fewer contraindications, CT myelography is CT with contrast is used when MRI is contraindicated but nowadays the use of CT has declined due to the efficiency of producing 3D images using EOS [48].

6.4.4 MRI Scan

MRI SCAN is a non-invasive method that uses a magnetic field for identifying tissue properties, by using numerous sequences comparing MRI to all other imaging techniques it's superior to visualize soft tissue and neural elements.

regardless of MRI's benefits there are limitations to its use too including its expensive cost limited availability and taking a long time it's not a first line choice, and the presence of implants causes artifacts and disturbs image analysis [48] also being a major Contraindications especially in the elderly's having lumbar scoliosis and also the presence of electrical conductive devices like intra cardiac defibrillators ICD, or other metallic implants such as cochlear implants, prosthetic valves and vascular stents, MRI are not used routinely in the assessment of isolated Lumbar scoliosis unless accompanied by a history or physical examination findings suggestive of neuropathy [49, 50]. MRI is also used in atypical cases of scoliosis like in (left thoracic scoliosis), in diagnosis of congenital curvature of spine [51]. Scoliosis in its self-causes some diseases in patients like syringomyelia [52], vertebral segmentation anomaly, intramedullary spinal tumor [53] or chiari malformation [54]. MRI is especially useful in young patients limiting unnecessary exposure to radiations, due to its expensive cost its use is limited to severe and congenital cases [55] a special method used in both MRI and CT scans [56] is by Rogers et al. [55] it's based on the intervertebral rotation of lumbar spine [56].

6.5 Treatment of Scoliosis

Factors affecting treatment options are Level of maturity of the patient's spine, is he fully developed or still growing?

The curvature parameters include degree, extent, its effect on daily life, site of the curve, and the possibility of progression.

Taking all those factors into account, any of the following treatment options may be recommended:

- Observation
- Exercises
- Bracing
- Surgery

6.5.1 Observation

In the beginning scoliosis doesn't have sign & symptoms that need surgery, the CNS corrects the abnormalities accordingly but as habituation occurs and prolonged deviation in alignment mechanisms of compensation try to restore balance but cause further deviations [57] it's necessary to slow down curve progression and not allow abnormal patterns of posture to develop by basic interventions like exercises and postural retaining [58]. In Adolescent Idiopathic Scoliosis: The eventual treatment aim is to keep the scoliosis of less than 50 ° at maturity, Observation is used when the curve is less than 25 ° without the need to take skeletal maturity into consideration, it consists of frequent radiographic examinations to detect curve advancements (5–6 ° changes in Cobb angle) ranging from 3 months to 6 months follow-ups, 3 monthly for patients with grade 0 or 1 Risser score (immature) with curve degrees around 25 and 6 monthly for patients with 3 or greater Risser score (mature) with curve degrees less than 20. In Early onset: Observation is for patients with low risk of progression of their curves, which are curves of less than 20 ° or less, follow up should be done 4–6 monthly, and another line of management should be started if the progression of the curve is more than 10 ° [59], the newest studies have a positive outlook on conservative management including outpatient physiotherapy consisting of exercises, postural training, and intensive rehabilitation and bracing [57]. Although successful but conservative management particularly bracing is involved with increased stress in patients and their parents due to its prolonged use extending months or years [58, 59].

6.5.2 Bracing

In patients with Adolescent idiopathic scoliosis bracing is recommended for patients who are Risser 2 or less with curves between 25–45 °. Braces aim to keep the curve from progressing and prevent it from reaching the surgical scale range at skeletal maturity, the thoracolumbar orthosis (TLSO) is the most commonly used brace, the type of brace used depends on the type of the curve [59]. Brace treatment is useful in lowering the curve progress to the surgical range and the benefits correlate with the duration spent wearing the brace [60]. In early onset scoliosis serial casting and bracing are two methods that are used in delaying or preventing curve progression. Serial casting has also been shown to cure some small idiopathic curves [61]. It is nonsurgical but still needs general anesthesia for its utilization and during routine changes every few months. It isn't well tolerated in patients with poor pulmonary function or with neuromuscular disorders. Bracing is a substitute for serial casting in early onset scoliosis in patients not able to tolerate the serial casting or step down from casting, its removable while casting isn't which may be an advantage or a reason for non-compliance [59].

6.5.3 Surgery

Not all scoliosis patients are responsive to conservative treatments in severe cases or progressive scoliosis the patient needs surgery. There are several indications of surgery generally using Cobb's method with curves more than 45–50 ° on the basis that:

Curves greater than 50 ° continue to progress even after skeletal maturity.

Greater curves affect pulmonary function and could even lead to respiratory failure.

Even surgery becomes difficult as the curve progresses.

Patient's wishes for surgery should be taken into consideration especially for curves in the gray zone that are of 45–50 ° [62].

The surgery can be divided into fusion and fusion less surgery. Fusion surgery are of 2 types [62].

Posterior instrumentation which has been the standard since its introduction by Paul Harrington [63] and anterior instrumentation which had been a choice for thoracolumbar ad lumbar scoliosis due to the fact that better correction can be made with shorter fusion levels. Fusion less surgery are done to control growth, to avoid fusion, to delay definitive fusion surgery or to increase thorax volume [62].

6.6 Complication of Scoliosis

Complication after surgical procedures of scoliosis occur like any other types of surgery, the compilations like:

Infection one of the most common complications after surgical procedures [64] especially infection of the surgical site more with gram positive organisms [65] also we have lung infections in form of pneumonia and sepsis or UTI, if we detect it early and manage it do rate of success if more than 85% [66, 67].

Neurological complications like bladder and bowel problems, visual disturbance, CVA, sensory and motor deficit, paralysis with different mechanism of the injury, and some patient with experience cauda equine syndrome, but majority of the patient have complete recover, but nearly %1 without recovery [68].

Bleeding: also, another complication occurs in most of the surgical procedures, more in those patients that's on aspirin [69].

The implants that are using during the correction or the surgery is the most common cause for repeating the operation, the complication include dislodgement, pain, malposition [70].

cardiopulmonary complications like cardiac arrest and heart failure, MI, early detection of the complication and treating them essential, with reduction of the risk factors like smoking and weight loss pre operatively increase the chance of the better outcome [71].

Vascular complications: DVT and pulmonary embolism occur in immobile patient especially after surgery and we need US of the leg for detecting it with D-dimer test and giving treatments.

Gastrointestinal complications like ileus occur after many surgical procured and early mobility is essential for treating these complications.

Genitourinary complications: UTI common post operative complications due to folly catheter, acute renal failure occur also due to hypo perfusion and dehydration, during the surgery damaging the nerve plexus of the spine with cause some complications like retrograde ejaculation so we should be careful [72].

6.7 Prevention

The prevention program for the scoliosis is important to prevent complication and early detection essential to put our focus on the prevention rather that treatment, and its done through the screening programs by scolio-meter to detect truncal rotation but its cost effective, when the large curves forms it accompany more complication [73].

Multiple Choice Questions

1. **In scoliosis spinal curvature with cobb angle more than ….. degree?**
   - A. 11
   - B. 10
   - C. 30
   - D. 6
2. **………………: is common condition in those disease that cause muscle hypotonia and contracture?**
   - A. Neuromuscular scoliosis
   - B. Idiopathic scoliosis
   - C. Congenital scoliosis
   - D. Asymmetry of the spine
3. **One of the simpler diagnostic procedures is the …………… that assesses posture and identifies scoliosis?**
   - A. Adams forward bend test
   - B. Risser test

C. Scoliosis test
D. Cub angel

4. **…………….: the most common symptoms in scoliosis?**

A. Neurological deficit
B. Leg pain
C. Deformity
D. Back pain

5. **The prevention program for the scoliosis is done through the screening programs by …………….. to detect truncal rotation?**

A. Scolio-meter
B. MRI
C. CT
D. X-ray

Answers
1. B
2. A
3. A
4. D
5. A

References

1. Aebi M. The adult scoliosis. Eur Spine J. 2005;14(10):925–48.
2. Van Goethem JW, Campenhout AV. Scoliosis. Spinal Imaging. 2007:95–108.
3. Ailon T, et al. Degenerative spinal deformity. Neurosurgery. 2015;77(Suppl 4):S75–91.
4. Carter OD, Haynes SG. Prevalence rates for scoliosis in US adults: results from the first national health and nutrition examination survey. Int J Epidemiol. 1987;16(4):537–44.
5. Arlet V, Odent T, Aebi M. Congenital scoliosis. Eur Spine J. 2003;12(5):456–63.
6. Hedequist D, Emans J. Congenital scoliosis: a review and update. J Pediatr Orthop. 2007;27(1):106–16.
7. Weinstein SL, Dolan LA, Cheng JC, Danielsson A, Morcuende JA. Adolescent idiopathic scoliosis. Lancet. 2008;371(9623):1527–37.
8. Cheng JC, Castelein RM, Chu WC, Danielsson AJ, Dobbs MB, Grivas TB, Gurnett CA, Luk KD, Moreau A, Newton PO, Stokes IA. Adolescent idiopathic scoliosis. Nat Rev Dis Primers. 2015;1(1):1–21.
9. Kearon C, Killian J. Fadors determining pulmonary function in adolescent idiopathic thoracic scoliosis. Am Rev Respir Dis. 1993;148:288–94.
10. Vialle R, Thévenin-Lemoine C, Mary P. Neuromuscular scoliosis. Orthop Traumatol Surg Res. 2013;99(1):S124–39.
11. Allam AM, Schwabe AL. Neuromuscular scoliosis. PM R. 2013;5(11):957–63.
12. Silva FE, Lenke LG. Adult degenerative scoliosis: evaluation and management. Neurosurg Focus. 2010;28(3):E1.
13. Youssef JA, et al. Current status of adult spinal deformity. Global Spine J. 2013;3(1):51–62.

14. Smith JS, Shaffrey CI, Berven S, Glassman S, Hamill C, Horton W, Ondra S, Schwab F, Shainline M, Fu KM, Bridwell K. Operative versus nonoperative treatment of leg pain in adults with scoliosis: a retrospective review of a prospective multicenter database with two-year follow-up. Spine. 2009;34(16):1693–8.
15. Dyck PE. The stoop-test in lumbar entrapment radiculopathy. Spine. 1979;4(1):89–92.
16. Smith AY, Woodside JR. Urodynamic evaluation of patients with spinal stenosis. Urology. 1988;32(5):474–7.
17. Weinstein SL. Health and function of patients with untreated idiopathic scoliosis. JAMA. 2003;289(20):2644.
18. Krishnan A, Dave BR, Kambar AK, Ram H. Coexisting lumbar and cervical stenosis (tandem spinal stenosis): an infrequent presentation. Retrospective analysis of single-stage surgery (53 cases). Eur Spine J. 2014;23(1):64–73.
19. Laslett M, Aprill CN, McDonald B, Young SB. Diagnosis of sacroiliac joint pain: validity of individual provocation tests and composites of tests. Man Ther. 2005;10(3):207–18.
20. Levin U, Stenström CH. Force and time recording for validating the sacroiliac distraction test. Clin Biomech. 2003;18(9):821–6.
21. Willen J, Danielson B. The diagnostic effect from axial loading of the lumbar spine during computed tomography and magnetic resonance imaging in patients with degenerative disorders. Spine (Phila Pa 1976). 2001;26(23):2607–14.
22. Yazici M, et al. Measurement of vertebral rotation in standing versus supine position in adolescent idiopathic scoliosis. J Pediatr Orthop. 2001;21(2):252–6.
23. Zetterberg C, et al. Postural and time-dependent effects on body height and scoliosis angle in adolescent idiopathic scoliosis. Acta Orthop Scand. 1983;54(6):836–40.
24. Maggio D, et al. Assessment of impact of standing long-cassette radiographs on surgical planning for lumbar pathology: an international survey of spine surgeons. J Neurosurg Spine. 2015;23:581–8.
25. Harzmann HC. Stellenwert Der Videorasterstereographie Als Schulärztliche Screeningmethode von Skoliotischen Fehlhaltungen Und Strukturellen Skoliosen. PhD Thesis, Ludwig-Maximilians-Universität, Medizinischen Fakultät, München, Germany, 2000.
26. Cobb RJ. Outline for study of scoliosis. Instructional course lectures. Am Acad Orthop Surg. 1948:261–75.
27. Komeili A, Westover LM, Parent EC, Moreau M, El-Rich M, Adeeb S. Surface topography asymmetry maps categorizing external deformity in scoliosis. Spine J. 2014;14:973–983.e2.
28. Langensiepen S, Semler O, Sobottke R, Fricke O, Franklin J, Schönau E, Eysel P. Measuring procedures to determine the Cobb angle in idiopathic scoliosis: a systematic review. Eur Spine J. 2013;22(11):2360–71.
29. Zhou GQ, Jiang WW, Lai KL, Zheng YP. Automatic measurement of spine curvature on 3-D ultrasound volume projection image with phase features. IEEE Trans Med Imaging. 2017;36(6):1250–62.
30. Pruijs JE, Hageman MA, Keessen W, van der Meer R, van Wieringen JC. Variation in Cobb angle measurements in scoliosis. Skeletal Radiol. 1994;23:517–20.
31. Chowanska J, Kotwicki T, Rosadzinski K, Sliwinski Z. School screening for scoliosis: can surface topography replace examination with scoliometer? Scoliosis. 2012;7:9.
32. Betsch M, Wild M, Jungbluth P, Thelen S, Hakimi M, Windolf J, Horstmann T, Rapp W. The rasterstereographic-dynamic analysis of posture in adolescents using a modified matthiass test. Eur Spine J. 2010;19:1735–9.
33. Kutanzi K, Lumen A, Koturbash I, Miousse I. Pediatric exposures to ionizing radiation: carcinogenic considerations. Int J Environ Res Public Health. 2016;13:1057.
34. Vainio H, Heseltine E, Wilbourn J. Priorities for future IARC monographs on the evaluation of carcinogenic risks to humans. Environ Health Perspect. 1994;102(6–7):590–1.
35. Balanov M, Howe G, Anspaugh L, Bouville A, Guskova A, Ivanov V, Kenigsberg J, Likhtarev I, Mettler F, Shore R, Thomas G. UNSCEAR 2008 report to the general assembly with scientific annexes volume II scientific Annexe B. Tech. rep; 2008.

36. Betsch M, Wild M, Jungbluth P, Thelen S, Hakimi M, Windolf J, Horstmann T, Rapp W. The rasterstereographic–dynamic analysis of posture in adolescents using a modified Matthiass test. Eur Spine J. 2010;19(10):1735–9.
37. Frobin W. Rasterstereography: a photogrammetric method for measurement of body surfaces. 2021.
38. Hackenberg L, Hierholzer E, Pötzl W, Götze C, Liljenqvist U. Rasterstereographic back shape analysis in idiopathic scoliosis after posterior correction and fusion. Clin Biomech. 2003;18(10):883–9.
39. Mangone M, Raimondi P, Paoloni M, Pellanera S, Di Michele A, Di Renzo S, Vanadia M, Dimaggio M, Murgia M, Santilli V. Vertebral rotation in adolescent idiopathic scoliosis calculated by radiograph and back surface analysis-based methods: correlation between the Raimondi method and rasterstereography. Eur Spine J. 2013;22(2):367–71.
40. Buzug, T.M. Computed tomography. In Springer handbook of medical technology; Krame, R., Hoffmann, K.P., Pozos, R.S.., Springer handbooks; Springer: Berlin/Heidelberg, 2011.
41. Brenner DJ, Hall EJ. Computed tomography—an increasing source of radiation exposure. N Engl J Med. 2007;357:2277–84.
42. Smith-Bindman R, et al. Radiation dose associated with common computed tomography examinations and the associated lifetime attributable risk of cancer. Arch Intern Med. 2009;169(22):2078–86.
43. Gocen S, Havitcioglu H, Alici E. A new method to measure vertebral rotation from CT scans. Eur Spine J. 1999;8(4):261–5.
44. Dubousset J. Three-dimensional analysis of the scoliotic deformity. The pediatric spine: principles and practice. 1994.
45. Ferguson AB. The study and treatment of scoliosis. South Med J. 1930;23(2):116–20.
46. Bunnell WP. Selective screening for scoliosis. Clin Orthop Relat Res. 2005;434:40–5.
47. Yawn BP, Yawn RA, Hodge D, Kurland M, Shaughnessy WJ, Ilstrup D, Jacobsen SJ. A population-based study of school scoliosis screening. JAMA. 1999;282:1427–32.
48. Rupp R, et al. Magnetic resonance imaging evaluation of the spine with metal implants. General safety and superior imaging with titanium. Spine (Phila Pa 1976). 1993;18(3):379–85.
49. Maiocco B, Deeney VF, Coulon R, Parks PF. Adolescent idiopathic scoliosis and the presence of spinal cord abnormalities. Spine. 1997;22:2537–41.
50. Do TMD, Fras CMD, Burke SMD, Widmann RFMD, Rawlins BMD, Boachie-Adjei OMD. Clinical value of routine preoperative magnetic resonance imaging in adolescent idiopathic scoliosis. J Bone Joint Surg. 2001;83:577–9.
51. Wright N. Imaging in scoliosis. Arch Dis Child. 2000;82(1):38–40.
52. Zhu C, Huang S, Song Y, Liu H, Liu L, Yang X, Zhou C, Hu B, Chen H. Surgical treatment of scoliosis-associated with syringomyelia: the role of syrinx size. Neurol India. 2020;68(2):299–304.
53. Shih RY, Koeller KK. Intramedullary masses of the spinal cord: radiologic-pathologic correlation. Radiographics. 2020;40(4):1125–45.
54. Bolognese PA, Brodbelt A, Bloom AB, Kula RW. Chiari I malformation: opinions on diagnostic trends and controversies from a panel of 63 international experts. World Neurosurg. 2019;130:e9–16.
55. Caro PA. Magnetic resonance imaging in children with scoliosis. Semin Musculoskelet Radiol. 1999;3(03):257–65.
56. Rogers B, Wiese S, Blankenbaker D, Meyerand E, Haughton V. Accuracy of an automated method to measure rotations of vertebrae from computerized tomography data. Spine. 2005;30(6):694–6.
57. Shakil H, Iqbal ZA, Al-Ghadir AH. Scoliosis: review of types of curves, etiological theories and conservative treatment. J Back Musculoskelet Rehabil. 2014;27(2):111–5.
58. Negrini S, Antonini G, Carabalona R, Minozzi S. Physical exercises as a treatment for adolescent idiopathic. A systematic review scoliosis. Pediatr Rehabil. 2003;6(3–4):227–35.

59. El-Hawary R, Chukwunyerenwa C. Update on evaluation and treatment of scoliosis. Pediatr Clin N Am. 2014;61(6):1223–41.
60. Weinstein SL, Dolan LA, Wright JG, Dobbs MB. Effects of bracing in adolescents with idiopathic scoliosis. N Engl J Med. 2013;369(16):1512–21.
61. Mehta MH. Growth as a corrective force in the early treatment of progressive infantile scoliosis. J Bone Joint Surg Br. 2005;87(9):1237–47.
62. Maruyama T, Takeshita K. Surgical treatment of scoliosis: a review of techniques currently applied. Scoliosis. 2008;3:6.
63. Harrington PR. Treatment of scoliosis. Correction and internal fixation by spine instrumentation. J Bone Joint Surg Am. 1962;44-A:591–610.
64. Schairer WW, Carrer A, Deviren V, Hu SS, Takemoto S, Mummaneni P, Chou D, Ames C, Burch S, Tay B, Sawyer A. Hospital readmission after spine fusion for adultspinal deformity. Spine. 2013;38(19):1681–9.
65. Abdul-Jabbar A, Berven SH, Hu SS, Chou D, Mummaneni PV, Takemoto S, Ames C, Deviren V, Tay B, Weinstein P, Burch S. Surgical site infections in spine surgery: identification of microbiologic and surgical characteristics in 239 cases. Spine. 2013;38(22):E1425–31.
66. Ahmed R, Greenlee JD, Traynelis VC. Preservation of spinal instrumentation after development of postoperative bacterial infections in patients undergoing spinal arthrodesis. Clin Spine Surg. 2012;25(6):299–302.
67. Sierra-Hoffman M, Jinadatha C, Carpenter JL, Rahm M. Postoperative instrumented spine infections: a retrospective review. South Med J. 2010;103(1):25–30.
68. Hamilton DK, Smith JS, Sansur CA, et al. Rates of new neurological deficit associated with spine surgery based on 108,419 procedures: a report of the scoliosis research society morbidity and mortality committee. Spine. 2011;36:1218–28.
69. Park HJ, Kwon KY, Woo JH. Comparison of blood loss according to use of aspirin in lumbar fusion patients. Eur Spine J. 2014;23(8):1777–82.
70. Smith JS, Klineberg E, Lafage V, Shaffrey CI, Schwab F, Lafage R, Hostin R, Mundis GM, Errico TJ, Kim HJ, Protopsaltis TS. Prospective multicenter assessment of perioperative and minimum 2-year postoperative complication rates associated with adult spinal deformity surgery. J Neurosurg Spine. 2016;25(1):1–4.
71. Sciubba DM, Yurter A, Smith JS, Kelly MP, Scheer JK, Goodwin CR, Lafage V, Hart RA, Bess S, Kebaish K, Schwab F. A comprehensive review of complication rates after surgery for adult deformity: a reference for informed consent. Spine Deform. 2015;3(6):575–94.
72. Shaffrey E, Smith JS, Lenke LG, Polly DW Jr, Chen CJ, Coe JD, Broadstone PA, Glassman SD, Vaccaro AR, Ames CP, Shaffrey CI. Defining rates and causes of mortality associated with spine surgery: comparison of 2 data collection approaches through the Scoliosis Research Society. Spine. 2014;39(7):579–86.
73. McCarthy RE. Prevention of the complications of scoliosis by early detection. Clin Orthop Relat Res. 1987;222:73–8.

Chapter 7
Spina Bifida

Ahmed Mostafa Abd-Elhady Elhagar and Zeinab Yousef Hashem

> Test your learning and check your understanding of this book's contents: use the "Springer Nature Flashcards" app to access questions using ▶ https://sn.pub/QCsfpd.
> To use the app, please follow the instructions in Chap. 1.

7.1 Introduction

Neurulation is a process of formation of neural tube which occurs during the third and fourth weeks after fertilization after stage of gastrulation. Neural tube is very important for formation and development of brain, spinal cord, meninges and part of spine around them [1].

Neurulation happens in many steps that started at the end of third week after fertilization by elevation of the lateral edges of ectoderm to form the neural fold and the depressed mid region between the lateral edges called neural groove. The whole layer then called neural plate of ectoderm [1, 2].

Neural plate is two parts the first one is the head which called the cranial end and the second part is the tail which called the caudal end. The cranial part will develop to form the brain and the caudal end will develop to form the spinal cord [3].

At week three the neural plate will give rise to the neural folds with depression in the midline that called neural groove. After fusion of the neural folds then the neural plate converts to neural tube which will develop to form brain and spinal cord [1, 2, 4].

A. M. A.-E. Elhagar (✉) · Z. Y. Hashem
GP, Fayoum University Hospital, Fayoum, Egypt
e-mail: am3477@fayoum.edu.eg; Zy1117@fayoum.edu.eg

K. F. AlAli, H. T. Hashim (eds.), *Congenital Spine Malformations*, https://doi.org/10.1007/978-3-031-59031-3_7

7.2 Definition of Spina Bifida

Spina bifida is a Latin word meaning split spine and it is a congenital disease that occurs due to abnormal neurulation and improper closure of the neural tube in the fourth week after fertilization and can affect the brain, spinal cord and spine according to the site of the lesion and severity of the disease.

7.3 Classification of Spina Bifida

7.3.1 Myelomeningocele

1:2/1000 of live births are diagnosed with myelomeningocele and risk increases to 2:3/1000 if myelomeningocele has been diagnosed in a previous birth, and 6:8/1000 after two births.

Myelomeningocele also known as spina bifida cystica or meningomyelocele is the most common and severe type of spina bifida that occurs due to the absence or incomplete formation of the vertebral arch and protrusion of meninges and spinal cord through this defect. This protrusion maybe covered by skin or not. The defect and protrusion can occur anywhere along the spinal axis, but the most common site is lumber region [1].

Myelomeningocele is considered a multifactorial disease genetic, environmental and other risk factors as maternal folic acid deficiency or Gestational Diabetes Mellitus. But there are many cases that are diagnosed with no apparent risk factor [5].

Most cases of myelomeningocele are not covered by skin. The absence of skin increases the risk of infection, which can lead to nerve destruction and sensory loss, paralysis, and orthopedic deformities [6].

Myelomeningocele is associated with hydrocephalus in 65:85% of patients and approximately 5: 10% of patients with myelomeningocele have clinically evident hydrocephalus at birth. And most patients with myelomeningocele have an associated Arnold Chiari type 2 syndrome [2, 3, 7].

7.3.2 Meningocele

Meningocele or Meningeal cyst is the least common type of spina bifida. It is due to a defect in the vertebral arch that leads to sac formation that formed due to protrusion of meninges without protrusion of spinal cord so this type is not usually associated with spinal cord damage or severe symptoms but babies who are diagnosed with meningocele may have minor problems [4].

The sacs are filled by CSF covered by dural and arachnoid membranes. The lumber spine and sacral regions are the commonest sites for posterior meningocele [8].

7.3.3 Spina Bifida Occuluta (SBO)

Occulta is a Latin word meaning hidden and Spina bifida occulta is the second most common and the mildest type of spina bifida, which usually occur due to a small defect in one or more of vertebrae due to the absence of a spinous process and a variable amount of lamina. The defect may be palpable or not. And the skin above it may be covered by hair, dimple or birth mark on the back over the site of the lesion and perhaps not. In spina bifida occulta there is no protrusion of meninges or spinal cord so spina bifida occulta is often asymptomatic and many patients aren't even aware they have it. And is often accidentally diagnosed later in life. Spina bifida occulta may be associated with lipoma, dermoid cyst, tethered cord, or diastematomyelia [9]. A systematic review studies found that there is no relation between spina bifida occulta and back pain. But there are other studies that suggest that spina bifida occulta is not always innocent and one study found that back pain severity increases in patients with spina bifida occulta [10–12].

7.3.4 Lipomyeloschisis (Dorsal Spinal Dysraphism)

In some cases, we found that spina bifida is associated with lipoma, Lipoma is a fibrous fatty tissue that extends through the spina bifida defect and connects to the spinal cord against the skin. There are many types of lipomyeloschisis, but the following three types are very important as they can lead to progressive neurological dysfunction:

1. Lipomyelomeningocele
2. Intra dural lipoma
3. Fibrolipoma of the filum terminale [13]

Before delving into the mechanism of lipomyeloschisis, we need to know that in embryonic development, the neural plate develops into a neural fold, which transforms into a neural tube, which in normal situations separates from the epidermal ectoderm by mesenchymal cells and that as a disjunction. After that, the neural tube will play the main rule in the formation of the brain and the spinal cord and mesenchymal cells in the formation of the structures will separate the spinal cord from the skin with epidermal ectoderm playing an important role in the formation [13].

In the case of early separation of the epidermal ectoderm that is called premature disjunction, leading to early invasion of the mesenchyme when the neural tube is not fully formed. Mesenchyme then develops into fat which disrupts the neural tube formation. When neural tissue doesn't become neural tube, we call it a neural placode and, in this case, we have a neural placode and a lipoma interface inside the spinal cord which is called lipomyelocele. But in case of lipomyelomeningocele the subarachnoid space enlarges and the make the meninges from outside the spinal cord so in lipomyelomeningocele the lipoma and neural placode are outside the spinal cord There is another type which is called intra dural lipoma and in this type neural type with mesenchyme are surrounded by dura so we call that intra dural lipoma [13].

In some cases spina bifida is associated with dermal sinus; we called that spinal dermal sinus. In spinal dermal sinus the tract starts at the skin surface and is usually located at either end of neural tube. The most common site of spinal dermal sinus is the lumbosacral area. This disease usually results from a failure of separation of cutaneous ectoderm from the neuro-ectoderm at the time of the neural groove closes [2].

7.4 Causes and Risk Factors of Spina Bifida

Neural tube defects which include mainly spina bifida malformation, occurs without a clear cause, but it is considered to be a multifactorial disease. Risk factors include genetic, nutritional and environmental factors or combination of any two or all of them [1]. Other rare cases can occur due to chromosomal errors, gene mutations, or teratogenic diseases [14].

7.4.1 Nutritional Factors

Many studies show that the lack of folic acid in the maternal diet during early pregnancy, especially from the fourth week of pregnancy to the 12th week of pregnancy, increases congenital anomalies. Neural tube defects and spina bifida in particular are linked to folic acid deficiency, but folic acid deficiency is not a definite cause of spina bifida, just a risk factor. Many cases occur without folic acid deficiency [15]. It has been proven that folic acid supplementation reduces the occurrence of neural tube defects from the first day of pregnancy until at least the end of the first 3 months of pregnancy. Folic acid intake can be supplemental or by eating fortified food [16]. Folic acid intake may reduce other congenital malformation like abruptio placenta and megaloblastic anemia [17].

When we intake folic acid which is the synthetic form that is converted in our body into the active form called tetrahydrofolate (THF) which is formed through a reduction process by the dihydrofolate reductase enzyme and then through an anther reduction process into 5-Methyltetrahydrofolate (5-MeTHF) will form, which is transformed to the blood and are absorbed by all cells, and due to the polyglutamation process, the folic acid polyglumate formed and cannot be exit from the cell. In cells, this form of folate contributes to the methylation process, purine and thiamine synthesis, and affects DNA synthesis. This rule of folic acid is very important in the formation of CNS neurotransmitters that affect the rapid process of growth in early pregnancy and closure of the neural tube formation. If the folic acid metabolism is disturbed or there is a deficiency, the neural tube defect or other malformation will occur [18].

7.4.2 Environmental Factors

Environmental risk factors are related to folic acid deficiency or suspicious metabolism.

- Antiepileptic drugs require folic acid for their hydroxylation action as a co-enzyme, these drugs interfere with the absorption of folic acid and alter the effect of folic acid by combative reaction leading to folic acid deficiency and incidentally affecting the neural tube formation [17].
- There are many other drugs affect folic acid metabolism and absorption and cause teratogenic effect as methotrexate, antacids, rifampicin, azathioprine, anti-malarial and anti-censer drugs [17, 18].
- Gestational Diabetes Miletus is associated with the occurrence of many comorbidities of the central nervous system, including neural tube defects, and hyperinsulinemia is an important risk factor for neural tube defects [17].
- Obesity in pregnancy is linked to the occurrence of neural tube defect, but the cause is unclear but may be due to the disruption in sex hormone levels and insulin resistance [17].
- Maternal smoking is associated with the occurrence of multicongenital abnormalities, including neural tube defects, since smoking reduces serum folate [17].
- Also vitamin B12 deficiency is considered one of the risk factors of neural tube defect occurrence due to its rule in neurotransmitters and neural receptors formation [17].
- Vitamin A intake during pregnancy cause teratogenic effect and neural tube defect [17].
- Polycyclic Aromatic Hydrocarbons: These are air pollutants that include organic materials such as coal, gasoline, oil, and wood. When pregnant women are exposed to air pollution from these organic agents, the risk of neural tube defects and spina bifida is 60%. This effect is not clearly explained, but it is expected that the polycyclic aromatic hydrocarbons decrease methylation of the DNA included in all infant cells [19].
- Arsenic poisoning and pesticides which accumulates in neuro-epthilial tissues of embryo and interfere with methylation process and DNA synthesis [19].
- Maternal hyperthermia especially in the first trimester cause many teratogenic and congenital anomalies as neural tube defect [19].
- There are many other factors may cause congenital anomalies and spina bifida like seizures, viruses, influenza, COVID19 vaccinations during pregnancy and several medications but there is no clear evidence prove that. These may link to maternal hyperthermia [19].

- There are environmental exposure cause mutations in some genes that influence methylation process and accordingly the folic acid pathway and DNA synthesis [19].

7.4.3 Genetic Factors

Genetic risk factors aren't a clear cause of spina bifida but are also associated with other environmental or nutritional risk factors [9].

There are variant gene mutation included in folic acid pathway may increase the risk of spina bifida like:

- 5, 10-methylenetetrahydrofolate (MTHFR)
- Methionine synthase (MTR)
- Methionine synthase reductase (MTRR)
- Methylenetetrahydrofolate dehydrogenase\ methylenetetrahydrofolate cyclohydrolase
- Folate receptor alpha (FR alpha)
- Folate receptor beta (FR beta)
- Reduced folate carrier
- Planar cell polarity (PCR)

There are more than 250 genes studied in humans and mice to be linked to spina bifida [9].

A family history of spina bifida or previous offspring with spina bifida from the same mother increases the risk of developing spina bifida and other congenital anomalies [1].

7.5 Clinical Presentation

Most spina bifida patients are diagnosed prenatally by ultrasound and have elevated alpha-fetoprotein levels, except for the mild and closed types. Mild cases of spina bifida may be asymptomatic and discovered only by investigations and radiology [1].

Spina bifida patients may present by neurological, urinary, and skeletal and mobility symptoms but the presentation varies by the severity and type [20].

Spina bifida infants may present with lethargy, poor feeding, irritability, stridor, or developmental delay when first presented. Older children present with back pain, cognitive and behavioral disorders, bowel dysfunction or orthopedic deformities [21].

The back appears with pilonidal sinus or sacs filled with spinal cord or CSF. In some cases, there is lipoma or swelling covered by normal skin. The position of the abnormality differs from types of spina bifida. Some cases presented with normal back skin and the condition discovered by radiological investigations [1, 21].

7.5.1 Neurological Manifestations

Most cases present with hydrocephalus as an association that needs urgent treatment, but we must rule out other causes of hydrocephalus. There are patients with Chiari type II malformation, which is characterized by compression of the brainstem or spinal cord. The symptoms can be apnea, laryngeal and pharyngeal paralysis, shortness of breath or nystagmus. Other cases may present with coordination and cognitive disorders [21].

The neurological abnormality depends on the type and severity of spina bifida. Neurological problems include:

Motor impairment, which varies with the level of the lesion, may be caused by upper and lower motor neuron lesion, may be asymmetric, may be associated with flaccid or spastic paralysis. Most patients have flaccid paralysis [21].

There are sensory affection and cranial nerves abnormality according to the type of the lesion. Coordination and cognitive disorders may occur with spina bifida [21].

Neurologic problems affect the stature and weight of children due to impairment and delay in growth and feeding problems.

Hydrocephalus may cause several complications as tethered spinal cord which presenting with scoliosis, pain and sensory affection, lower brainstem affection, syringomyelia and cranial nerves dysfunction [20, 21].

7.5.2 Orthopedic Manifestations

The orthopedic complications differ according to the level of spinal cord affection. If the lesion is thoracic or lumber, there are lumber lordosis, knee and hip contracture and flexion, equinus contractures of the ankles and genu valgus.

If the level is sacral, there are many knee and foot abnormalities, lumber lordosis and hip contractures [21].

Urinary complications:

Many cases of spina bifida have urinary complications as neurogenic bladder, urine incontinence, urine retention, kidney dysfunction and anatomical disorders. Most cases need catheterization from the first 24 h after delivery [20].

There are other complications related to any association of spina bifida like chromosomal or congenital abnormalities.

After treatment procedures, many symptoms improve but the neurologic and orthopedic complication do not resolve completely. The spina bifida patient's life is difficult and need many rehabilitation methods to cope with their condition.

They showed developmental delay for their ages, need special care to do some motor, sensory, cognitive and behavioral disorders [1, 21].

7.5.3 Signs

By examination, we may find the signs of increase the intracranial tension, sensory, motor and autonomic signs according to site of the lesion and severity of the disease.

7.6 Diagnosis

7.6.1 Prenatal Screening and Diagnosis

Prenatal screening is very useful and important for diagnosing spina bifida and other neural tube defects, which requires parents to decide whether to complete or terminate the pregnancy. These screening tests are very important and routine for women with a family history of spina bifida or a history of previous offspring with spina bifida or anencephaly. Diagnosis is very important for perpetration to appropriate care [1].

Alpha-Fetoprotein (AFP)

Marked elevation amniotic fluid alpha-fetoprotein concentration is considered a screening test to rule out, but not detect, spina bifida or other neural tube defects. Alpha-fetoprotein is measured by amniocentesis assay in the second trimester of pregnancy, and peak concentration in the 13th to 15th weeks. If the concentration increases, we suspect neural tube defects, especially spina bifida and anencephaly. Alpha fetoprotein is elevated in 70–75% of cases. Skin covered myeloceles are unlikely to be detected by measurement of alpha fetoprotein. Also, we need more tests to prove the diagnosis [1].

Assay of acetylcholinesterase in the amniotic fluid also required for the diagnosis of neural tube defects. It can be measured after increasing alpha-fetoprotein concentration [22].

Ultrasonography

Regular maternal and fetal ultrasonography during pregnancy is the non-invasive diagnostic method of neural tube defect especially open spina bifida and anencephaly. The closed types covered by skin or lipoma can't be identified during pregnancy [1].

Sonography identifies the fetal spine by examining the sagittal, coronal, and axial planes from the first trimester through the end of pregnancy. Ultrasound identifies the spina bifida sacs and the neural tissue they contain. Through ultrasound we can identify other features such as small biprital diameter for gestational age and other abnormalities in the spine that associated with spina bifida.

Through the second trimester we can use ultrasound to diagnose and follow up the severely of spina bifida and other anomalies [1].

Most cases of spina bifida have specific sonographic features that are specific and diagnostic for spina bifida:

- Lemon sign: It refers to the loss of convexity of the frontal bone and occurs with slight flattening, which is noted between 16 and 24 weeks of pregnancy, but after that it may not reappear [1, 22].
- Banana sign: refers to shape of the cerebellum that appears with downward traction. Also, it can't appear after 24th week of pregnancy [1, 22].

Also, we can detect hydrocephalus and its severity, venteiculomegally and other spinal and cranial abnormality which associated with spina bifida [1].

Once spina bifida is diagnosed, we search for renal, cardiac and any organic anomalies [22].

Urine analysis and culture, and kidney function tests in form of urea and creatinine at birth to evaluate renal function in neonates with spina bifida is very important. and in case of presence of symptoms or signs of UTI or in cases of vesicoureteral reflux then you need to do regular bacterial urinary cultures so as urology consultation is very important [1].

Post-natal Diagnosis and Investigation

MRI and CT can be used to diagnose and measure the severity of spina bifida and any spinal abnormalities to help determine appropriate treatment. They are used to assess hydrocephalus. They also give an indication of the prognosis of the cases. They can also be used for aftercare after surgical procedures. After diagnosis of spina bifida, renal ultrasound, karyotyping, echocardiography and bowel imaging are preformed to detect associated anomalies [1, 22].

7.7 Prevention

Prevention is better than cure. The incidence of myelomeningocele has undergone a significant reduction which is due to the good and accurate prenatal diagnosis and the option of early pregnancy termination. The utilization of folic acid in periconceptual phase as there are a lot of studies that demonstrating that there is reduction in the incidence of spina bifida with folic acid supplementation .it is important to do more studies about genetic factors that play role in spina bifida as it may plays an important role in prevention the incidence of spina bifida [23].

7.8 Management

7.8.1 Pre-natal Management

In case of diagnosing of open spina bifida during pregnancy, we can perform surgery during pregnancy to repair malformation before birth. Some studies said that treatment of open spina bifida before birth may reduce the need to drain fluid away from brain with a shunt after birth. But at the same time this surgery can increase the risk of preterm labor. The technique of surgery is the same after birth but before birth the surgery is performed by making a small opening in the uterus in med pregnancy to access the fetus and close spina bifida [1, 23].

7.8.2 Post-natal Management

In many places the standard care for spina bifida is antibiotic, sac closure and ventriculoperitoneal shunt in case of presence hydrocephalus and can be implemented in the perinatal in around 93:95% of patients. In cases with irreparable sac or active infection of bleeding the supportive care can be the main treatment [24].

A good medical history and examination are very important steps in knowing if there are any associated congenital diseases or complications. So, motor specifically, we should assess the motor function of the lower extremities. Assessing sensation and autonomic function are also very important [24].

Orthopedic examination and consultation are very important to exclude any deformities. And urinary bladder catheterization and urological consultation also is very important [24, 25].

Steps of Lesion Management

Surgical treatment should occur within the first 48 h and is preferred within the first 24 h unless there is a contraindication to surgery, as early treatment reduces the risk of infection, which increases when the defect closed after the first 36 h. It is important to know that early closure of myelomeningeocele defect is not associated with improvement of neurological function.

1. First step of treating the defect is to know how big the defect is
2. Then if the defect is ruptured or not like in case of ruptured lesion, the antibiotic will be necessary and we should give antibiotic as gentamicin
3. Cover the lesion with Telfa then with sponges soaked in normal saline or Ringer's lactate and form a ring of sterile gauze around the lesion if it is cystic or protruding to prevent desiccation

4. Then put the patient prone (Trendelenburg position) to keep the pressure off the lesion [2, 24, 25].
5. In case of myelomenangiocele defect:

In Patient without hydrocephalus must doctors wait at least 3 days after defect repair before shunting but in cases with hydrocephalus myelomenangiocele repair and shunting may be performed in the same sitting to avoid the incidence of infection as possible as we can

Surgical Technique of Myelomeningocele Repair

After prevention of desiccation. Don't allow chemical substances as antimicrobial and scrub solutions to contact neural placode and don't use monopolar cautery and finally at every point during the closure avoid placing tension on the neural placode.

After general anesthesia the baby's position should be prone position with head slightly lower than the back which is very important as it prevents that the cerebrospinal fluid will not be replaced by air. Then the site of surgery should be cleaned well and the myelomeningocele should be washed by warm sterile saline and the surrounding skin by betadine or hibiclens. You should be careful that betadine and hibicens should not be placed on placode as they are neurotoxic. Draping of anus is the next step with a generous area exposed so that good skin flaps can be mobilized [2, 26].

Midline linear incision is performed at the upper limit of defect over the spinous processes of the first two normal vertebrae above apex of the defect and then the incision extended along the border between the arachnoid that cover the defect and the skin around them and circumferentially until the entire placode is completely freed, saving the skin is very import to be used in the final reconstruction of the superficial layers, finally the linear incision is made at the lower extremity of defect .

Identification of normal dura rostral to defect is very important for the safe dissection.

After incision the next step is placode dissection from the surrounding arachnoid which is usually starts at the upper limit of defect and proceeds circumferentially along the borders and then followed be section of the filum termiale which is usually found under the most caudal part of placode and this procedure is important to minimize the risk of 2ry tethering.

Good inspection of intradural space is very important to make sure there is no other abnormality as lipoma or dermoids [23, 26].

After dissection of placode, the placode will be at the bottom of dural sac. The next step it will be the neural tube reconstruction to this end. The edges of placode will be in the midline and pia-arachnoid borders are sutured under microscope magnification with 7–0 non absorbable monofilament [26].

After neural tube reconstruction, the next step is reconstruction of dural sac. After identified the intact meningeal at the upper part of malformation just below the first normal vertebra where the malformed dura continues into the normal dural sac from this point the dural layer is dissected along the borders of defect proceeding centripetally from the periphery to the midline. Isolation of dura is very difficult at the edge of malformation as it is the side where there is fusion between the dura and thoracolumbar fascia so dissection should start at midline. The newly developed dural sheets are approximated on the midline and sutured by 5–0 silk suture or monofilament. And we can do double layer suture in case of very large dural flap. During dural closure you should avoid making compression on any neural structures. When the dural sheets appears insufficient Dural patching can be performed using different dural substitutes as fascia or muscle in this case we can use the thoracolumbar fascia, putting the fascial flap between the incomplete dural sheets and suture it to cover the dural defect [2, 26].

If the patient's anatomy doesn't allow using autologous grafting, we can use allografts as cadaveric dura or silicon. The new dural substitute composed only of colloidal collagen (TissuDura) which is have low risk of development of inflammatory response which made it be used beside that the patch ensures that there is adequate dural closure. Dural closure should be water-tight as it protects against CSF leakage that may happen postoperative or CSF pooling at the site of surgery which will lead to delay healing of spinal wound and increase the risk of complication. Reinforcement of dural closure by suturing the thoracolumbar fascia over the reconstructed dural sac is very important. After dural closure the next step is subcutaneous and skin mobilization and closure [2, 23, 26].

7.8.3 Post-operative Management

Bladder catheterization regimen.

Delay occipital-frontal head circumference. Measurement.

Avoid narcotics to avoid risk of respiratory depression.

If there is no shunt, keep the patient flat to decrease CSF pressure on incision with regular ultrasonography of head [2, 23].

Multiple Choice Questions

1. **All of the following are types of spina bifida except:**

   A. Spina bifida occulta
   B. Meningocele
   C. Hemophilia
   D. Myelomenigocele

   Answer: C. Hemophilia

2. **Surgical treatment of spina bifida can be done before birth**

   A. Yes
   B. No

   Answer: A. Yes

3. **Which of the following is a complication of spina bifida?**

   A. Hydrocephalus
   B. Depression
   C. Orthopedic deformities
   D. Urinary bladder affection
   E. All of the above

   Answer: E. All of the above

4. **A person with spina bifida can't fully participate in life**

   A. Yes
   B. No

   Answer: B. No

5. **Do people with spina bifida always have mental health problem?**

   A. Yes
   B. No

   Answer: B. No

6. **Folic acid can reduce the risk of having spina bifida**

   A. Yes
   B. No

   Answer: A. Yes

7. **What is the meaning of spina bifida?**

   A. Sealed spine
   B. Split spine
   C. Forked spine

   Answer: B. Split spine

8. **Patient with spina bifida always require pre-medication before dental treatment**

   A. Yes
   B. No

   Answer: B. No

9. **There is always no skin cover the defect**

   A. Yes
   B. No

   Answer: B. No

10. **What is the difference main between myelomeningocele and myelocele**

   A. Presence or absence of a subcutaneous mass
   B. Exposure of a neural placode through a midline skin defect

C. Position of neural placode relative to skin surface
D. Presence or absence of a dilated central canal

Answer: C. Position of neural placode relative to skin surface

11. **The neural plate bends and folds to form the neural tube during which stage**

A. Primary neurulation
B. Secondary neurulation
C. Gastrulation

Answer: A. Primary neurulation

References

1. Copp AJ, Adzick NS, Chitty LS, Fletcher JM, Holmbeck GN, Shaw GM. Spina bifida. Nat Rev Dis Primers. 2015;1:15007. https://doi.org/10.1038/nrdp.2015.7.
2. Greenberg M. Handbook of neurosurgery. 9th ed. 2013.
3. Van Speybroeck A, Beierwaltes P, Hopson B, McKee S, Raman L, Rao R, Sherlock R. Care coordination guidelines for the care of people with spina bifida. J Pediatr Rehabil Med. 2020;13(4):499–511. https://doi.org/10.3233/PRM-200738.
4. Spina bifida fact sheet. National Institute of Neurological Disorders and Stroke. https://www.ninds.nih.gov/Disorders/Patient-Caregiver-Education/Fact-Sheets/Spina-Bifida-Fact-Sheet. Accessed 28 Aug 2019.
5. Hebert L, Hillman P, Baker C, Brown M, Ashley-Koch A, Hixson JE, Morrison AC, Northrup H, Au KS. Burden of rare deleterious variants in WNT signaling genes among 511 myelomeningocele patients. PLoS One. 2020;15(9):e0239083. https://doi.org/10.1371/journal.pone.0239083.
6. Hunter AGW, Cleveland RH, Blickman JG, Holmes LB. A study of level of lesion, associated malformations and sib occurrence risks in spina bifida. Teratology. 1996;54:213–8. https://doi.org/10.1002/(SICI)1096-9926(199611)54:5<213::AID-TERA1>3.0.CO;2-0.
7. Kim I, Hopson B, Aban I, Rizk EB, Dias MS, Bowman R, Ackerman LL, Partington MD, Castillo H, Castillo J, Peterson PR, Blount JP, Rocque BG. Decompression for chiari malformation type II in individuals with myelomeningocele in the national spina bifida patient registry. J Neurosurg Pediatr. 2018;22(6):652–8. https://doi.org/10.3171/2018.5.PEDS18160.
8. Chellathurai A, Kathirvelu G, Mukkada PJ, Rajendran K, Ramani R. Spinal dysraphisms: a new anatomical-clinicoradiological classification. Indian J Radiol Imaging. 2022;31(4):809–29. https://doi.org/10.1055/s-0041-1741100.
9. Mohd-Zin SW, Marwan AI, Abou Chaar MK, Ahmad-Annuar A, Abdul-Aziz NM. Spina bifida: pathogenesis, mechanisms, and genes in mice and humans. Scientifica. 2017;2017:5364827. https://doi.org/10.1155/2017/5364827.
10. van Tulder MW, Assendelft WJ, Koes BW, Bouter LM. Spinal radiographic findings and nonspecific low back pain. A systematic review of observational studies. Spine. 1997;22(4):427–34. https://doi.org/10.1097/00007632-199702150-00015. PMID 9055372. S2CID 41462354.
11. Taskaynatan MA, Izci Y, Ozgul A, Hazneci B, Dursun H, Kalyon TA. Clinical significance of congenital lumbosacral malformations in young male population with prolonged low back pain. Spine. 2005;30(8):E210–3. https://doi.org/10.1097/01.brs.0000158950.84470.2a. PMID 15834319. S2CID 21250549
12. Avrahami E, Frishman E, Fridman Z, Azor M. Spina bifida occulta of S1 is not an innocent finding. Spine. 1994;19(1):12–5. https://doi.org/10.1097/00007632-199401000-00003.

13. Mehta DV. Magnetic resonance imaging in paediatric spinal dysraphism with comparative usefulness of various magnetic resonance sequences. J Clin Diagn Res. 2017;11(8):TC17–TC22. https://doi.org/10.7860/JCDR/2017/30134.10393.
14. Mitchell LE, Adzick NS, Melchionne J, Pasquariello PS, Sutton LN, Whitehead AS. Spina bifida. Lancet. 2004;364(9448):1885–95. https://doi.org/10.1016/S0140-6736(04)17445-X. PMID: 1555566
15. Greene ND, Stanier P, Copp AJ. Genetics of human neural tube defects. Hum Mol Genet. 2009;18(R2):R113–29. https://doi.org/10.1093/hmg/ddp347.
16. Oumer M, Tazebew A, Silamsaw M. Birth prevalence of neural tube defects and associated risk factors in Africa: a systematic review and meta-analysis. BMC Pediatr. 2021;21(1):190. https://doi.org/10.1186/s12887-021-02653-9.
17. Kondo A, Matsuo T, Morota N, Kondo AS, Okai I, Fukuda H. Neural tube defects: risk factors and preventive measures. Congenit Anom. 2017;57:150–6. https://doi.org/10.1111/cga.12227.
18. Blom HJ, Shaw GM, den Heijer M, Finnell RH. Neural tube defects and folate: case far from closed. Nat Rev Neurosci. 2006;7(9):724–31. https://doi.org/10.1038/nrn1986.
19. Isaković J, Šimunić I, Jagečić D, Hribljan V, Mitrečić D. Overview of neural tube defects: gene-environment interactions, preventative approaches and future perspectives. Biomedicines. 2022;10(5):965. https://doi.org/10.3390/biomedicines10050965.
20. Alriksson-Schmidt AI, Thibadeau JK, Swanson ME, Marcus D, Carris KL, Siffel C, Ward E. The natural history of spina bifida in children pilot project: research protocol. JMIR Res Protoc. 2013;2(1):e2. https://doi.org/10.2196/resprot.2209.
21. Vinck A, Nijhuis-van der Sanden MWG, Roeleveld NJA, Mullaart RA, Rotteveel JJ, Maassen BAM. Motor profile and cognitive functioning in children with spina bifida. Eur J Paediatr Neurol. 2010;14(1):86–92. https://doi.org/10.1016/j.ejpn.2009.01.003.
22. Gober J, Thomas SP, Gater DR. Pediatric spina bifida and spinal cord injury. J Personal Med. 2022;12(6):985. https://doi.org/10.3390/jpm12060985.
23. Caldarelli M, Rocco C, Özek M, Cinalli G, Maixner W. Myelomeningocele primary repair surgical technique. 2008. https://doi.org/10.1007/978-88-470-0651-5_10.
24. Hettige S, Shtaya A, Gangopadhyay AN, Bifida S. Handbook of pediatric surgery; 2022. p. 343–50. https://doi.org/10.1007/978-3-030-84467-7.
25. Radcliff E, Cassell CH, Laditka SB, et al. Factors associated with the timeliness of postnatal surgical repair of spina bifida. Childs Nerv Syst. 2016;32:1479–87. https://doi.org/10.1007/s00381-016-3105-3.
26. Myelomeningocele repair. Barrow Quarterly. 2000 16(4).

Chapter 8
Spinal Canal Stenosis

Ahmed Hassan A. Rady, Emry Atwa Ibrahim Mansour, and Mohammedbaqer Ali Al-Ghuraibawi

Test your learning and check your understanding of this book's contents: use the "Springer Nature Flashcards" app to access questions using ▶ https://sn.pub/QCsfpd.
To use the app, please follow the instructions in Chap. 1.

Spinal stenosis is a medical term in which there is a narrowing of the spinal canal and foramina that houses the neural structures. The term "spinal canal stenosis" was introduced by the neurosurgeon Henk Verbiest in 1954, stenosis can affect variable parts of the spine such as the cervical, thoracic, and lumbar. For males, it is common to be affected by the cervical spine and thoracic spine, while the lumbar spine is more common in females. Generally, spinal canal stenosis can be either congenital or acquired [1].

8.1 Lumbar Spinal Stenosis

Lumbar spinal canal stenosis is defined by a narrowing of the canal, which compresses the Dural sac and nerve roots. Lumbar stenosis can be either congenital or acquired, rarely the stenosis occurs congenitally (9% of patients), while the acquired form is more common [2]. The typical presentation of spinal stenosis is seen in patients in their 50 s and 60 s and presented with neurogenic claudication,

A. H. A. Rady (✉) · E. A. I. Mansour
Faculty of Medicine, Ain Shams University, El Weili, Egypt

M. A. Al-Ghuraibawi
Faculty of Medicine, University of Warith Al-Anbiyaa, Karbala, Iraq

K. F. AlAli, H. T. Hashim (eds.), *Congenital Spine Malformations*,
https://doi.org/10.1007/978-3-031-59031-3_8

radiculopathy, or mechanical back pain. Nowadays, it is mostly diagnosed in patients above 65 years old. Its main mechanism is a tightening of the spinal canal or could be due to relative movements of the vertebrae with the spine, which then leads to compression of the canal and/or foraminal space. L3–L4 and L4–L5 are the most common sites of stenosis at the disc level, L2–L3 and L5–S1 are less common. The midsagittal diameter of the lumbar canal is more than 13 mm [3].

When stenosis occurs, the anteroposterior canal diameter becomes between 10 mm and 13 mm, and if the diameter of the anteroposterior is less than 10 mm, this presentation is called absolute stenosis. Another indicator for stenosis is sac diameter, which normally should be more than 100 mm. in a condition of spinal stenosis, the sac is compressed and it measures between 76 mm and 100 mm when the stenosis is moderate, and less than 76 mm in severe cases [3].

8.2 Pathology of Lumbar Spine Stenosis

Normally the spine column works accurately with all its structures, spine, disc, bone, and ligaments. To maintain the appropriate spine motions and mechanics. At the time of birth, disc surfaces are composed of 50% nucleus pulposus and 50% of annulus fibrosus. As age increases, the chondrocytes replace the notochordal cells of the nucleus pulposus, and also water amount within the disc will decrease. Collagen type II with age will be more than type I collagen, then the collagen fibers within the nucleus are increased. As we get older, the spinal disc undergoes many changes in collagen, water content, and proteoglycan metabolism [4, 5]. The concentration of chondroitin 4-sulfate and chondroitin 6-sulfate decreases while the keratin sulfate to chondroitin sulfate ratio increases. These changes lead to a condition where the disc has fewer abilities to resist axial loading, leading to microscopic alterations that progress to visible degeneration over time. As the spinal disc is dehydrated, clefts can be identified in the central portion of the nucleus pulposus, which migrate toward the peripheral annular fibrosis and plate [6]. This can result in annular tears, bulging of the disc, and focal extrusions. In addition, the vascular supply of the disc decreases with age, and nutrition occurs through the end plate and outer annular diffusion. And facets bear up to 25% of the axial load. Lumbar spinal stenosis can be presented in many parts of the spine as the cervical canal (between the dotted lines in the lateral zone, and outside those lines), lateral recess, and foramen [7].

The vertebral bodies approximate and the neuroforamen experiences a decrease in vertical height as the disc height decreases. This leads to redistribution of stress, with posterior loads shifting to the facet joints. Increased stress in the facet joints leads to capsular synovitis, cartilage thinning, and eburnation, leading to facet degeneration, increased segmental motion, and osteophyte formation [8].

Osteophytes are a manifestation of facet hypertrophy leading to neuroforamen and central canal narrowing. In normal status, the exiting nerve occupies 305 of the neuroforamen, but if disc height decreases it results in radiculopathy symptoms [9]. In conclusion, the risk of spinal canal compression and symptoms of claudication, and radiculopathy are caused by disc collapse and the formation of osteophytes [10].

Lumbar spinal stenosis also involves ligamentum flavum buckling and hypertrophy. This ligament is quite thin in children, but it gets thick as the intervertebral height decreases, this hypertrophy is associated with ossification and proliferation of chondrocytes, hyalination of collagen fibers, calcium crystal deposition, and a proliferation of collagen type II. Some patients may have a compression due to epidural fat [11, 12].

8.3 Typical Presentation of Lumbar Spinal Stenosis

Lumbar spinal stenosis presents with discomfort in the legs, back, or both. Varying in severity. It can lead to cauda equina syndrome in severe cases represented by sudden pain and loss of bowel and bladder function. Lower limb pain due to lumbar spinal stenosis can result from nerve dysfunction caused by vascular issues. Blocked nerve roots can lead to pain, dysfunction, reduced function, and neurogenic claudication [13–15].

Cauda equina syndrome is an extreme form causing low back pain, sciatica, saddle anesthesia, motor weakness, and incontinence. It is recommended that the treatment be within 2 days of presentation. Patients with spinal stenosis can be asymptomatic or may present with a wide range of symptoms making the management more challenging. Symptoms include pain due to osteophytes, ligaments, or disc material pressing on the canal. Along with symptoms that may persist or worsen. Unfortunately, there is not enough historical data on this condition, so the information is mostly provided by surgeons' experiences and empirical studies. Following 2–5 years after presentation, about 20% of patients may worsen with non-operative treatment, while about 40% remain the same, and the other 40% get better [16, 17].

8.4 Approach to the Patient with Lumbar Spinal Stenosis

Depending on the exact underlying cause, the patient may exhibit different symptoms. 80% of patients have leg pain, while 65% of patients have back pain. Often the patient is not pinpointed accurately. As we discussed above, stenosis can be congenital or acquired, congenital stenosis patients are divided into idiopathic or developmental subtypes. Secondary stenosis may experience claudication and radicular symptoms, as seen in achondroplasty dwarfs. However, there are only a few people present with stenosis caused by a congenital predisposition. It is more common for patients to have a developmentally narrowing canal, leading to a higher susceptibility to compression of the root when spondylitis changes occur [17].

The majority of patients with spinal stenosis are diagnosed with acquired stenosis, and degenerative or spondylosis is the most common type. Degenerative stenosis is classified into two, static or dynamic. Static degenerative stenosis is mainly due to any factor narrowing the canal as a disc bulge, while dynamic degenerative stenosis is caused by the relative motion of the spinal elements. It is important to know that there are many systemic illnesses that may lead to the narrowing of the spinal canal such as diabetes, Paget's disease, and pseudogout. We can differentiate symptoms if they are neurogenic or mechanical symptoms by that mechanical symptoms are associated with back pain, while neurogenic symptoms are characterized by neurologic claudication or radiculopathy [18, 19]. Patients who have spondylolisthesis are affected by central canal stenosis. Pain is poorly localized, it begins with the gluteal region, thigh, and calf.

As the condition progresses, patients have increased pain and paresthesia with ambulation and extension, and eventually develop a classic neurogenic pattern. Often lying spine, flexion, sitting, or squatting will relieve symptoms. Severe cases present weakness, rest pain, neurogenic bladder, and cauda equina syndrome. It is critical to differentiate between neurogenic claudication and vascular claudication by the proper examination and history taken from patients [20]. Cramping or sensation of tightness that progresses from distal to proximal, are characteristics of vascular diseases, whereas neurogenic claudication is associated with sharp discomfort with numbness that progresses from proximal to distal. We can differentiate between these two etiologies by the Bicycle versus treadmill test, when patients get pain in both tests that means it is vascular, while when patients tend to do well on the bicycle and have more discomfort on the treadmill test it indicates the neurogenic case. Another diagnostic test is up-hill versus down-hill walking, uphill walking forces patients to lean forward, which increases the spinal canal space and provides relief for stenotic patients. Conversely, walking downhill will result in an extension of the lumbar spine and is less tolerable for patients with spinal stenosis. Vascular claudication patients often feel better walking uphill.

During the physical examination, it is important to conduct a comprehensive evaluation of the patient's strength, sensation, and reflexes. A good observation of patients walking can help in detecting any unusual limping. Evaluation also includes an assessment of distal pulses, upper extremity reflexes, and cervical examination to exclude cervical spine issues. In addition, the hip should be rotated to rule out osteoarthritis as a potential source of pain, vascular cases are associated with absent pedal pulses along with atrophic changes in the nails of their lower extremities [21, 22].

8.5 Investigations and Tests for Lumbar Spinal Stenosis

Plain radiographs, magnetic resonance imaging (MRI), myelography/computed tomography (CT)-myelography, Bicycle/treadmill test, vascular studies (arterial Doppler/ultrasound), electrodiagnostic studies (electromyography and nerve conduction studies).

8.6 Palin Radiographs

Lumbar spinal stenosis is mostly seen at the level L4–L5 vertebrae, next most common site is L3–L4 followed by L5–S1.

To do a proper evaluation of the lumbar spine, multiple radiographic views should be obtained, including at minimum anteroposterior, lateral, and flexion-extension views, and Ferguson view and oblique may be helpful. For identifying nerve compression between the sacral ala and the L5 transverse process, the Ferguson view is particularly helpful. We may observe a narrow interpedicular distance on an anteroposterior view in patients with congenital stenosis, spondylosis changes, and cyst formation. Endplate osteophytes and benign vertebral sclerosis may seen anteriorly, while from a posterior view, we observe discrete osteophytes, which may project into lateral recess or anteromedially, causing central stenosis. Large claw osteophytes or traction spurs may be observed also in cases of instability [23].

8.7 Magnetic Resonance Imaging

MRI is useful for detecting the changes in the nucleus and can measure the water content of the disc.

Increased proton signal on T2-weighted images—As hydrated nucleus pulposus.
Degeneration disc—Dark, isointense signal.
Free fluid in annular tears and fissures—Increased T2 signal.
Degenerative disc disease—Radial tears.
MRI can also reveal potential facet degeneration via increased fluid seen in the facet joint on axial imaging.
Due to the ability of MRI to allow direct sagittal imaging and to provide a contrast between fat, nerve roots, and epineural vessels, it is the best modality to detect lateral compression, when we observe an obliterated fat in the entire foramen we diagnose nerve root compression. About 30–50% of asymptomatic adults have abnormal MRI findings. Many advantages in MRI including its non-invasive nature and an 87.6% correlation with surgical findings [24, 25].

8.8 CT-Myelography

It was first performed in 1976. This technique is used mainly to identify spinal canal stenosis if MRI is contraindicated for any reason, or when dynamic imaging is required. CT is a very useful tool to evaluate spinal stenosis as it offers good details compared to plain films. It provides multiple plane view images, axial, coronal, and sagittal; making its advantages for our purposes. Patients with spinal stenosis will exhibit a canal that appears more triangular and less oval, due to the prominent articular pillars which create a trefoil shape. Keep in mind that these changes are normal in 10–20% of patients at the level of L5–S1. Nerve root sleeve compression can be diagnosed with obliteration of the fat plane around the nerve [26].

In patients with suspected congenital stenosis, pedicle length can be measured. CT has an 83% correlation with surgical findings. It is invasive providing image study of the central and lateral canals. Overall, it can detect lumbar stenosis as a ventral extradural defect due to disc bulges or end plate osteophytes. An hourglass constriction of the thecal sac is an appearance of central stenosis [27].

Technique: In CT myelography the water-soluble non-ionic iodination contrast should be used with a 3 g maximum dose to avoid neurotoxicity.

- 10 mL of 300 mg iodine/mL in cervical CT myelography.
- 15–17 mL of 240 mg iodine/mL in whole spinal CT myelography.
- 15–17 mL of 180 mg iodine/mL in lumbar spine CT myelography.

Now it is more common for the use of CT fluoroscopy for a CT, guided lumbar puncture (is. Initially patient status with fluoroscopy then transported to CT). It is recommended that patients should be rolled many times before CT image acquisition and high-resolution thin slices (0.5–0.625 mm).

8.9 Complications of CT Myelography

1. Complications related to lumbar puncture such as infection, bleeding, and post-lumbar puncture headache.
2. Rarely there is an iodinated contrast media allergy.
3. Rarely there are seizures.
4. Injection of the spinal cord or conus medullaris.

8.10 Bicycle/Treadmill Tests

Progressive spinal stenosis patients may experience symptoms such as cramps discomfort, paresthesia, and lower limb pain, which are present in a patient with vascular claudication, so to distinguish between neurogenic claudication and vascular claudication we use the bicycle and treadmill test [28].

During the bicycle test, spinal stenosis patients' symptoms worsen when a patient is upright due to limited space in the lateral sac. This challenge can be circumvented by bending forward during the bicycle test. On the other hand, in vasculogenic claudication patients may face difficulties in both tests (bicycle and treadmill tests).

8.11 Electrodiagnostic Testing

When there is peripheral neuropathy and potential symptoms, using electromyography (EMG) and nerve conduction velocity (NCV) are useful in the diagnosis. It is the main investigative modality for suspected myopathy patients. For patients with risk factors such as diabetes mellitus or a non-classic history of neurogenic claudication, electrodiagnostic testing becomes necessary for the diagnosis of spinal stenosis [28–30].

8.12 EMG Limitations

1. Recording is affected by adipose tissue.
2. Surface EMG measures only superficial muscles.
3. Less effective in children, infants, patients with paralysis, and unresponsive patients. Because of the velocity activation of muscles in needle EMG.

8.12.1 Diagnosis of Lumbar Spinal Stenosis

Presentation of lumbar spinal stenosis may be confused with other diseases, such as musculoskeletal diseases (including hip and knee arthritis, pelvis or sacral disorder, and external compartment syndrome), vascular conditions (such as peripheral vascular disease or abdominal aorta aneurysm), neurologic disorders (diabetic and peripheral neuropathy, cervical myelopathy, amyotrophic lateral sclerosis, multiple sclerosis (MS), meralgia paresthetica, common peroneal entrapment, tarsal tunnel syndrome), and others (renal disorders, retroperitoneal tumor, depression or somatization disorders, and other psychiatric disorders), litigation, and psychosocial [31].

To differentiate between lumbar spinal stenosis and all these conditions, a proper history and examination must be performed. And using all the techniques that we discussed above.

8.13 Treatment

Treatment of spinal canal stenosis can be surgical or non-surgical, depending on a specific case, presentation, and condition.

Non-surgical treatment: in some rare cases, we better start with non-surgical treatment, including NSAID (non-steroidal, anti-inflammatory drugs), physical therapy treatment, heat therapy, cryotherapy, transcutaneous electrical nerve stimulation, traction, bracing, ESI (epidural steroid injection), SNRB (selective nerve root block).

Surgical treatment: unsuccessful, non-surgical treatment is an indication to start the surgical management [32].

Indications for surgery: Functional limitations that affect walking tolerance and daily activities, and intractable pain, as in neurogenic claudication with lower limb pain.

If the patient has isolated back pain surgery is less successful.

It is important to strike a balance between potential iatrogenic instability and adequate decompression during decompression, which will be done accurately if surgeons are fully aware of anatomy [32].

8.14 Surgical Techniques Used in Lumbar Spinal Stenosis

- Central laminectomy.
- Laminectomy with lateral recess and foraminal decompression.
- Laminoplasty.
- Posterior spinal fusion with and without decompression.
- Internal body fusion (anterior lumbar interbody fusion, posterior lumbar interbody fusion, and transform lumbar interbody fusion)

8.15 Central Laminectomy

- Laminectomy with lateral recess and foraminal decompression.
- Laminoplasty.
- Posterior spinal fusion with and without decompression.
- Interbody fusion (anterior lumbar interbody fusion, posterior lumbar interbody fusion, and transforaminal lumbar interbody fusion).

8.16 Central Laminectomy

It is the gold standard procedure for decompression in treating lumbar spinal stenosis. The patient is placed in a prone position on the operating table. The chest and pelvis are padded while the abdomen is kept free; the surgeon makes a vertical incision then the lumbodorsal fascia is dissected, followed by subperiosteal dissection by a Cobb elevator and electrocautery. The beginning of this procedure is by exposing the spinous process and then dissecting down into the lamina. To confirm the correct level we use plain radiographs or/and fluoroscopy for the desired decompression [32].

Hemostatic methods and techniques must be achieved to minimize any surgical complications. Using a Leksell rongeur to remove the inferior half of the spinous process at the top of the decompression and the superior half of the spinous process of the inferior level to be decompressed. A surgeon should identify the ligament flavum, and dissect the insertion of the ligament from the undersurface of the inferior edge of the most caudal lamina, that is where central decompression begins. As the decompression is extended laterally to the pedicle, the protection of the dura should be provided by an angled Dural elevator. On each side, at least 50% of the facet joints should be preserved when fusion is not planned.

To do a sufficient decompression of the nerve root entrance zone, medial facetectomy and removal of osteophytes ridge adjacent to the intervertebral disc space. Additionally, to the previous steps, it is important to maintain as much of the pars interarticularis as possible. If there is a protruding or extruded disc that is compressing the exiting nerve root, discectomy is necessary. Fortunately, the success rate is typically very high in this procedure.

8.17 Laminectomy with Lateral Recess Decompression and Foraminotomy

It is crucial to completely decompress the lateral recess. The anatomical area that is below the pedicle and anterior to the pars requires careful undercutting of the hypertrophic facet joints. Moreover, it is important to avoid total facetectomy because it can lead to iatrogenic segmental instability. It is recommended to visualize the nerve root and thecal sac while undercutting into the neuroforamen and lateral recess to prevent injury of the dura or nerve root. The nerve root should be identified to ensure potency and is followed through the neuroforamen and a probe passed in a direction parallel to the nerve root can be used. Overall, it is very effective and has a high success rate.

8.18 Laminoplasty

It is a technique with wide use for decompression of multilevel stenosis in the cervical region. In lumbar spinal stenosis, it is often used for central and lateral decompression while preserving the posterior osseous architecture. This involves removing the interspinous ligaments with a rongeur, exposing the interlaminar space then placing the lamina spreader against the spinous process. Before completing laminoplasty, on the medial 20% of the Facet joints and the inner one-third of the lamina, an osteotomy is performed.

8.19 Posterior Spinal Fusion

Cases of instability at the involved motion segment, degenerative scoliosis, revision decompression at the same level, resection of more than 50% of the facets bilaterally, and degenerative spondylolisthesis. In these cases, Arthrodesis may be necessary. It is important to preserve at least 50% of the facet joint if only compression without instrumentation is planned. Always remember that removing too much bone laterally can cause a fracture, segmental instability, and pain.

8.20 Interbody Fusion

Interbody fusion used to treat motion segment pain since the mid-twentieth century, and it was preferred over posterolateral fusion because of the potential for bony fusion by Wolff's law, which is increased when placing a bone graft in the anterior and middle spinal column to receive a good blood supply more than the posterolateral elements, further promoting bony fusion.

ALIF (anterior lumbar interbody fusion), TLIF (transforaminal lumbar interbody fusion), and PLIF (posterior lumbar interbody fusion). Their use can lead to longer surgery time, more blood loss, and a high risk of complications post-surgically and during the surgery.

8.21 Interspinous Devices

Used for treating lumbar spinal canal stenosis and other lower back pain. The purpose of these devices is to induce lumbar flexion by separating the lumbar spinous processes, which rehabilitates height and leads to the thickened ligamentum flavum tightening, widening of the central canal, and expanding of neural exit foramen. These devices have the capacity to relieve stress on the facet joints and enhance spinal stability.

8.22 Indications to Use Interspinous Devices

- Neurogenic claudication due to lumbar stenosis, which is relieved with flexion that has failed conservative treatment.
- Rescue treatment in a condition of recurrent neurogenic claudication syndrome following laminectomy, spinal stimulator implantation, or adjacent segment degeneration.
- Spondylolisthesis (in its first degree).

- Intervertebral lower back pain.
- Non-traumatic instability.
- Facet syndrome.

Contraindications: Depending on a specific case, there are many conditions that the interspinous device is contraindicated; these include:

- Low back pain that doesn't radiate to the groin, gluteal, or lower limb.
- Previous decompression at the targeted level, or spinal fusion.
- Severe hypertrophy of facet joints that requires resection which leads to instability.
- Grade 2 of spondylolisthesis.
- Spondylolysis, severe scoliosis, and osteoporosis.

Complications: About 15% of patients will experience a wound complication, 5% of them may get spinous process fracture, 4% may experience device loosening, breakage, or migration, and only 1% will have a deep infection.

Approximately 33% of patients will develop new or worsening pain and there are 15% may require re-operation.

Multiple Choice Questions

1. **A 49-year-old female complains of lumbalgia at the L5–S1 level with irradiation to the lower limb. The condition had been evolving for around 2 years, despite conservative therapy consisting of non-steroidal anti-inflammatory drugs, muscle relaxants, physiotherapy, and analgesia. The patient had no history of trauma. MRI was conducted showing disc bulging, facet joint hypertrophy, and yellow ligament which caused the narrowing of the canal. According to this case presentation, all the following are correct except:**

   A. We should start surgical treatment if the non-surgical succussed.
   B. Interspinous devices are contraindicated in this case.
   C. If the patient experienced difficulties in both bicycle and treadmill tests, that indicates the vascular cause.
   D. The suspected diameter of the anteroposterior is less than 10 mm.
   E. The region of stenosis is not the most common among other types of lumbar stenosis.

2. **The following are complications of CT myelography except:**

   A. Complications related to lumbar puncture such as infection, bleeding, and post-lumbar puncture headache.
   B. Seizures.
   C. Iodinated contrast media allergy.
   D. Injection of the spinal cord or conus medullaris.
   E. Paralysis.

3. **Interspinous device contraindications include all the following except:**
    A. Grade 2 of spondylolisthesis.
    B. Previous decompression at the targeted level.
    C. Facet syndrome.
    D. Severe hypertrophy of facet joints that requires resection which leads to instability.
    E. Low back pain that doesn't radiate to the groin, gluteal, or lower limb.
4. **According to the Technique In CT myelography which of the following is correct:**
    A. To avoid neurotoxicity the maximum dose of iodine is 10 g.
    B. 10 mL of 300 mg iodine/mL in lumbar spine CT myelography.
    C. 15–17 mL of 240 mg iodine/mL in lumbar spine CT myelography.
    D. 15–17 mL of 180 mg iodine/mL in lumbar spine CT myelography.
    E. 30–80 mL of 240 mg iodine/mL in lumbar spine CT myelography.
5. **All the following are Indications to use interspinous devices except:**
    A. Rescue treatment in a condition of recurrent neurogenic claudication syndrome following laminectomy, spinal stimulator implantation, or adjacent segment degeneration.
    B. Spondylolisthesis (in its first degree).
    C. Intervertebral lower back pain.
    D. Non-traumatic instability.
    E. Grade 2 of spondylolisthesis.

References

1. Arbit E, Pannullo S. Lumbar stenosis: a clinical review. Clin Orthop Rel Res. 2001;384:137–43.
2. Atlas SJ, Delitto AN. Spinal stenosis: surgical versus nonsurgical treatment. Clin Orthop Rel Res. 2006;443:198–207.
3. Bassewitz H, Herkowitz H. Lumbar stenosis with spondylolisthesis. Current concepts of surgical treatment. Clin Orthop Rel Res. 2001;384:54–60.
4. Bono CM, Lee CK. Critical analysis of trends in fusion for degenerative disc disease over the past 20 years: influence of technique on fusion rate and clinical outcome. Spine. 2004;29(4):455–63.
5. Chad DA. Lumbar spinal stenosis. Neurol Clin. 2007;25:407–18.
6. Bridwell KH, Sedgewick TA, O'Brien MF, et al. The role of fusion and instrumentation in the treatment of degenerative spondylolisthesis with spinal stenosis. J Spinal Disord. 1993;6(6):461–72.
7. Gibson JN, Waddell G. Surgery for degenerative lumbar spondylosis: updated. Cochrane Rev Spine. 2005;30(20):2312–20.
8. Grob D, Hunke T, Dvorak J. Degenerative lumbar spinal stenosis: decompression with and without arthrodesis. J Bone Joint Surg Am. 1995;77(7):1036–41.

9. Haig AJ, Geisser ME, Tong HC, et al. Electromyographic and magnetic resonance imaging to predict lumbar stenosis, low back pain and no back symptoms. J Bone Joint Surg Am. 2007;89:358–66.
10. Herkowitz HN, Kurz LT. Degenerative lumbar spondylolisthesis with spinal stenosis: a prospective study comparing decompression with decompression and intertransverse process arthrodesis. J Bone Joint Surg Am. 1991;73(6):802–8.
11. Hilibrand AS, Rand A. Degenerative lumbar stenosis: diagnosis and management. JAAOS. 1999;7:239–49.
12. Jenis LG, An HS. Spine update: lumbar foraminal stenosis. Spine. 2000;25:889–94.
13. Kirkaldy-Willis WH, Wedge JH, Yong-Hing K, Reilly J. Pathology and pathogenesis of lumbar spondylosis and stenosis. Spine. 1978;3(4):319–28.
14. Kostuik JP, Harrington I, Alexander D, et al. Cauda equina syndrome and lumbar disc herniation. J Bone Joint Surg Am. 1986;68(3):386–91.
15. Mardjetko SM, Connolly PJ, Shott S, Degenerative lumbar spondylolisthesis. A meta-analysis of literature 1970–1993. Spine. 1994;19(20 Suppl):2256S–65S.
16. Patel C, Truumees, Gitlin J, Herkowitz H. Symptomatic spinal stenosis adjacent to a previous lumbar fusion. Presented at NASS 17th Annual Meeting; October 30, 2001; Montreal, QC, Canada.
17. Postacchini F. Spine update: surgical management of lumbar spinal stenosis. Spine. 1999;24:1043–7.
18. Weinstein JN, Lurie JD, Tosteson TD, et al. Surgical versus nonsurgical treatment for lumbar degenerative spondylolisthesis. N Engl J Med. 2007;356(22):2257–70.
19. Weinstein JN, Tosteson TD, Lurie JD, et al. Surgical versus nonsurgical therapy for lumbar spinal stenosis. N Engl J Med. 2008;358(8):794–810.
20. Whitecloud TS III, Davis JM, Olive PM. Operative treatment of the degenerated segment adjacent to a lumbar fusion. Spine. 1994;19(5):531–6.
21. Zdeblick TA. A prospective, randomized study of lumbar fusion. Spine. 1993;18(8):983–91.
22. Tan SB. Spinal canal stenosis. Singapore Med J. 2003;44(4):168–9.
23. Melancia JL, Francisco AF, Antunes JL. Spinal stenosis. Handb Clin Neurol. 2014;119:541–9. https://doi.org/10.1016/b978-0-7020-4086-3.00035-7.
24. Cowley P. Neuroimaging of spinal canal stenosis. Magn Reson Imaging Clin N Am. 2016;24(3):523–39. https://doi.org/10.1016/j.mric.2016.04.009.
25. Van Goethem JWM, van den Hauwe L, Parizel PM. Spinal imaging: diagnostic imaging of the spine and spinal cord. Springer; 2010.
26. Postacchini F. Management of lumbar spinal stenosis. J Bone Joint Surg Br. 1996;78-B(1):154–64. https://doi.org/10.1302/0301-620x.78b1.0780154.
27. Mayo Foundation for Medical Education and Research. Spinal Stenosis. Mayo Clinic. 2022. Retrieved September 17, 2022, from https://www.mayoclinic.org/diseases-conditions/spinal-stenosis/symptoms-caues/syc20352961#:~:text=Spinal%20stenosis%20happens%20when%20the,spinal%20stenosis%20have%20no%20symptoms.
28. Messiah S, Tharian AR, Candido KD, Knezevic NN. Neurogenic claudication: a review of current understanding and treatment options. Curr Pain Headache Rep. 2019;23(5):32.
29. Urits I, Burshtein A, Sharma M, Testa L, Gold PA, Orhurhu V, Viswanath O, Jones MR, Sidransky MA, Spektor B, Kaye AD. Low back pain, a comprehensive review: pathophysiology, diagnosis, and treatment. Curr Pain Headache Rep. 2019;23(3):23.
30. Bagley C, MacAllister M, Dosselman L, Moreno J, Aoun SG, El Ahmadieh TY. Current concepts and recent advances in understanding and managing lumbar spine stenosis. F1000Res. 2019;8:F1000 Faculty Rev-137.
31. Melancia JL, Francisco AF, Antunes JL. Spinal stenosis. Handb Clin Neurol. 2014;119:541–9.
32. Johnsson KE, Rosen I, Uden A. The natural course of spinal stenosis. Clin Orthop Rel Res. 1992;279:82–6.

Chapter 9
Dorsal Enteric Fistula

Ateeba Kamran

> Test your learning and check your understanding of this book's contents: use the "Springer Nature Flashcards" app to access questions using ▶ https://sn.pub/QCsfpd.
> To use the app, please follow the instructions in Chap. 1.

9.1 Introduction

Dorsal enteric fistula is a combined anterior and posterior spinal deformity due to splitting of the notochord secondary to the failure of the dissolution of the connection between the endoderm and the ectoderm forming an endo–ectodermal fistula. The fistula opens at the dorsal aspect of the embryo in association with a gastrointestinal anomaly and rarely a urogenital abnormality [1].

9.2 Classification

Dorsal enteric fistulas are classified as spinal defects anatomically, specifically as closed neural tube defects. Embryologically the disorder is attributed to defective gastrulation thus being classified as a disorder of notochord integration.

A. Kamran (✉)
Karachi Medical and Dental College, Karachi, Pakistan

K. F. AlAli, H. T. Hashim (eds.), *Congenital Spine Malformations*,
https://doi.org/10.1007/978-3-031-59031-3_9

The lesions of the split notochord syndrome can be divided into two broad categories: visceral malformations and central nervous and spinal malformations. Dorsal enteric fistulas are visceral malformations [2, 3]. Visceral malformations also include posterior enteric sinuses, diverticula, and cysts.

9.3 Embryogenesis and Pathophysiology

The embryo develops with a primary notochord defect. The persistence of the endoderm-ectoderm connection is the main culprit which results in the splitting of the notochord. Thus, the malformation leads to abnormal development of the neurenteric canal, notochord, and para-axial mesoderm forming the spinal column which can be attributed to the defect [4].

9.3.1 Formation of the Neurenteric Canal

Towards the end of the second week, the embryonic disc has a bilaminar configuration. At the beginning of the third week, the primitive streak spans over the caudal half on the dorsal aspect of the embryo on the surface of the epiblast [5]. Elongation of the primitive streak continues caudally while the proliferation of its cephalic end establishes the primitive node (Hensen's node).

Invagination occurs when cells migrate towards the primitive streak from the epiblast and slide under it. Following invagination, displacement of the hypoblast occurs due to some of the migrating cells. This forms the endoderm. Others settle between the newly formed endoderm and the epiblast to form the mesoderm. The ectoderm is formed by the remaining epiblast cells [6].

The process of the formation of the notochord begins when the prenotochordal cells, embedded in the primitive node, migrate cranially through the primitive streak. These cells lodge into the hypoblast to form the notochordal plate. With the displacement of the hypoblast and incoming endoderm cells, the notochordal plate detaches from the endoderm forming the notochord. In addition to the notochord, the cells from the primitive node migrate laterally giving rise to the paraxial mesoderm [7].

The notochord extends caudally to the primitive pit, which is found at the cephalic end of the streak in the region of the primitive node. The neurenteric canal forms here, specifically where the primitive pit forms an indentation in the epiblast.

The neurenteric canal brings forth a connection between the amniotic cavity and the yolk sac (primitive intestinal cavity). Normally, this canal degenerates when the development of the notochord is complete however its persistence leads to the splitting of the notochord. This phenomenon is the basis of many theories [7].

9.3.2 Theories

Multiple theories have been put forward to explain the embryogenesis of the split notochord syndrome.

A.O. Kovaleski, a Russian pathologist, put forward the theory that the persistence of the neurenteric canal induces the split notochord syndrome. However, variability in the location of the defect and association of visceral anomalies were questions that remained unanswered [7].

Bremmer et al. suggested that the adhesion between the endoderm and ectoderm leads to the presence of an accessory neurenteric canal which attributes to the connection between the gut and dorsal midline structures. The degree of involvement is dependent on the abnormal migration of the Hensen's node.

Pang D. further expanded on Bremmer's postulation that the adhesion may get surrounded by the condensation of mesenchyme forming an endomesenchymal tract.

According to Beardmore and Wigglesworth, incomplete separation of the endoderm and the ectoderm may cause adhesions within the primitive streak. The endodermal-ectodermal adhesion may interfere with the process of invagination and midline integration of the mesoderm between the ectoderm and the endoderm. The adhesion may form an endomesenchymal tract. This is an accessory neurenteric canal. During the formation of the notochord, the developing structure would have to bifurcate around it causing dissection of the notochord.

According to Saunders et al. in 1943, a primary midline notochordal integration defect leads to secondary changes occurring in the paraxial mesoderm which results in a split notochord. The connection between the primitive intestine and the notochord is not completely terminated post the split. A medial interosseous space is created. The endoderm and the primitive gut herniate through this space, consequently adhere to the dorsal ectoderm and ultimately rupture out (Fig. 9.1).

Stevenson et al. proposed that vascular compromise could lead to disruption in the region of the neural folds which results in the failure of the closure of neural tubes.

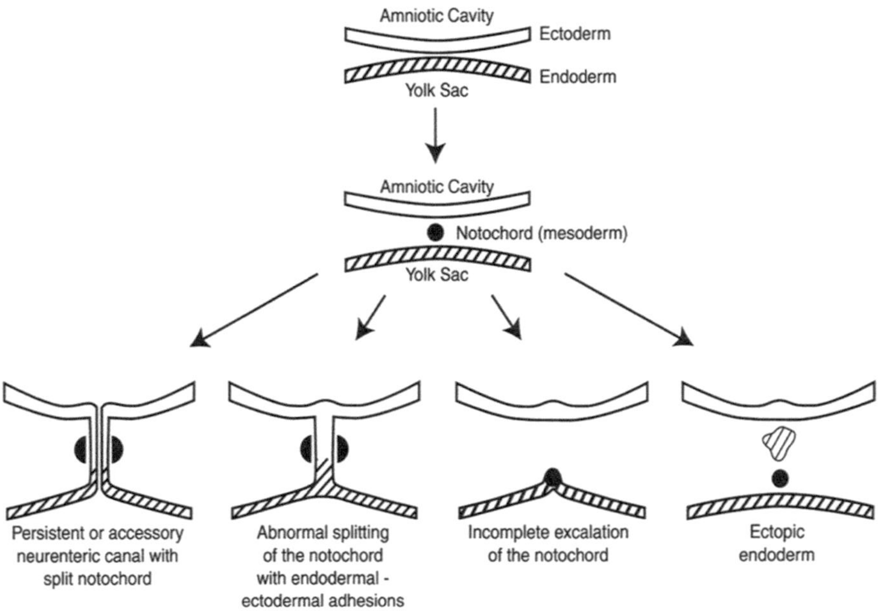

Fig. 9.1 Schematic diagram of the theories of pathogenesis representing the spectrum of neurenteric malformations including the persistent neurenteric canal with a split notochord and endodermal-ectodermal adhesions. (Adapted from Baek W, Lachkar S, Iwanaga J, et al. (September 28, 2018). Comprehensive Review of Spinal Neurenteric Cysts with a Focus on Histopathological Findings. Cureus 10(9): e3379. https://doi.org/10.7759/cureus.3379. https://www.cureus.com/articles/14161-comprehensive-review-of-spinal-neurenteric-cysts-with-a-focus-on-histopathological-findings)

9.4 Clinical Features

The retained link between the ectoderm and the endoderm leads to a dorsal enteric fistula. The fistula, along with its contents, course through the prevertebral soft tissue, the vertebral bodies, and the spinal canal. Involution or fibrosis of any portion of this tract may give rise to a fistula or cyst.

Visceral malformations comprise the posterior enteric remnants which include the mesenteric or posterior mediastinal duplications, cysts, or diverticula. A fibrous connection (a stalk) is the source of attachment of the posterior enteric remnants to the vertebral body anteriorly. The vertebral body may be bifid. The presence of a complete ventral and dorsal spina bifida is unusual.

Histopathological examination of the posterior enteric remnant reveals that its walls contain smooth muscles and enteric mucosa with columnar epithelium however variation may be present in the epithelium in the wall adjacent to it with no indication of its origin due to its flat or atrophic appearance. Broncho-pulmonary or other tissues originating predominantly from the developing gut are occasionally seen.

9.5 Types of Posterior Enteric Remnants

1. Posterior enteric fistulae: If the embryonic fistula fully persists due to failed obliteration, then a tract starting from the gut passes through the mesentery or the mediastinum and a complete spina bifida (which may be accompanied by a diplomyelia or diastematomyelia) is present. It terminates on the skin of the back, with an opening in the midline.
2. Posterior enteric sinus: Only the dorsal (posterior) portion of the embryonic fistula is intact. A sinus running forward to the midline of the skin of the back is present. It forms from the enteric or cutaneous tissues. A posterior or complete spina bifida may exist.
3. Posterior enteric diverticula: The ventral (anterior) portion of the embryonic fistula persists only. It is connected to the bowel. There is a risk of bowel strangulation or rotation in these patients. A fibrotic adhesion to a vertebral body may form. An anterior or complete spina bifida may be present.
4. Posterior enteric cyst: The intermediate or midline portion of the embryonic fistula or diverticulum is present only. These are found in the intraspinal or paraspinal compartments. They may be pre-vertebral, vertebral, or post-vertebral in position, the latter having been labeled as teratomatous cysts. A combined, ventral, or dorsal spina bifida may exist (Fig. 9.2).

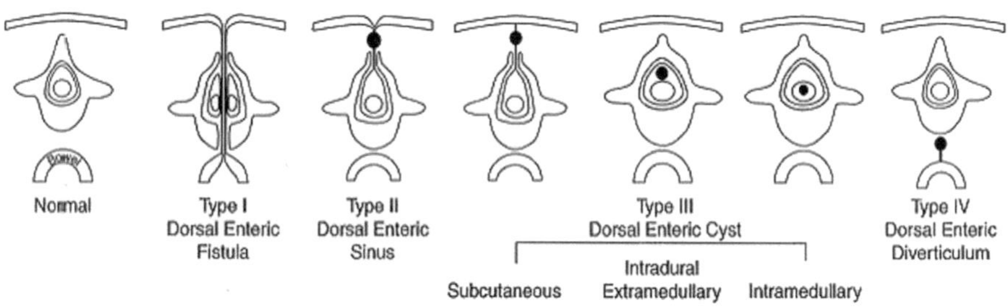

Fig. 9.2 Bentley and Smith classification of the posterior enteric remnants including the dorsal enteric fistula. (Adapted from Baek W, Lachkar S, Iwanaga J, et al. (September 28, 2018). Comprehensive Review of Spinal Neurenteric Cysts with a Focus on Histopathological Findings. Cureus 10(9): e3379. https://doi.org/10.7759/cureus.3379. https://www.cureus.com/articles/14161-comprehensive-review-of-spinal-neurenteric-cysts-with-a-focus-on-histopathological-findings)

9.6 Presentation

The presentation of the anomaly at different stages is as follows:

1. At birth, communication is present between the bowel and the dorsal skin forming a bowel ostium. Neonates present with meconium coming out of the opening at the back. This condition is very severe and is the gravest presentation.
2. An early presentation will reveal an obstruction or infection of the gastrointestinal tract and meningitis.
3. A delayed presentation will consist of a neurenteric cyst that is infected and has formed an abscess. Intraspinal enteric cysts are seen in the age group between 20 and 40 years of age which may present as episodic local or radicular pain that may eventually lead to myelopathy. If it is accompanied by a tethered cord or diastematomyelia, progressive neurological pathology can ensue.

   It impacts both males and females. The location of the fistula varies in every case. They are most commonly seen in the colon (large intestine). They may also occur in either the distal ileum or cecum. Along with gastrointestinal malformations, urogenital and anorectal defects may also be present (Fig. 9.3).

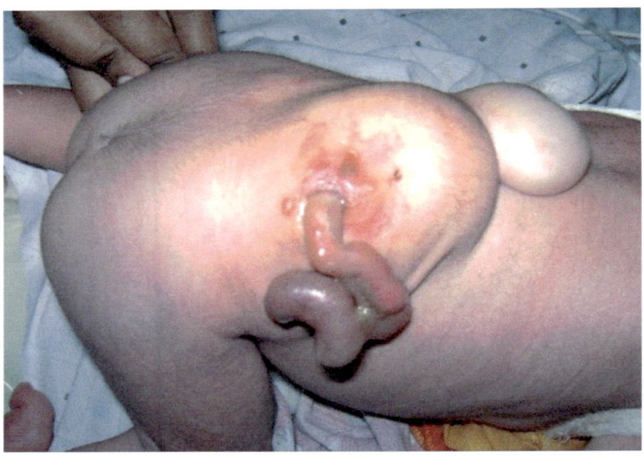

Fig. 9.3 A neonate presenting with a meningomyelocele (the cystic swelling over the lumbosacral area that is covered with skin) along with a dorsal enteric fistula (the intestine-like structure present at the peak of swelling). (Adapted from Srivastava, P., Gangopadhyay, A. N., Gupta, D. K., & Sharma, S. P. (2010). Split notochord syndrome associated with dorsal neuroenteric fistula: A rare entity. Journal of Pediatric Neurosciences, 5(2), 135–137. https://doi.org/10.4103/1817-1745.76112. https://www.ncbi.nlm.nih.gov/pmc/articles/PMC3087992/)

9.7 Neuroimaging

Radiography will aid in assessing the presence and magnitude of vertebral clefting. A follow-up with CT/MR imaging is required to determine the level of fistulation and the degree of cyst involvement. The cervicothoracic spine is mostly involved and occasionally involvement of the lumbosacral spine is seen.

9.8 Management

Every case of the dorsal enteric fistula is managed differently. It is based on the specific anomalies and systems involved and these vary from case to case. Thus management is individualized based on the presenting scenario. These cases are usually referred to pediatric surgeons more than neurosurgeons due to their presentation notably involving the bowel.

If a cyst is present then incision and drainage will be required. This should be followed by a pathological assessment. This is mandatory to rule out infection.

Complete surgical excision is the best treatment. Cystic material can cause arachnoiditis. This can cause surgical difficulty if operations are delayed due to the formation of dense adhesions.

A colostomy is performed with complete excision of the fistula. It is essential to prevent spinal cord contamination. To prevent further neurological decline, the spinal defect is closed. If the spinal cord is tethered, it is untethered.

Multiple Choice Questions

1. **The neurenteric canal forms in the region of the**:

   A. Hypoblast
   B. Primitive pit
   C. Yolk sac
   D. Amniotic cavity

2. **Posterior enteric remnants include all of the following except**:

   A. Diverticulum
   B. Sinus
   C. Cyst
   D. Diastematomyelia

3. **The following statement concerns the posterior enteric fistula**:

   A. The embryonic fistula is fully intact
   B. The dorsal part of the embryonic fistula is intact
   C. The ventral part of the embryonic fistula is intact
   D. The intermediate part of the embryonic fistula is intact

4. **A neonate with a dorsal enteric fistula will present at birth with**:

   A. Meconium coming out of the bowel ostium cranially
   B. Meconium coming out of the bowel ostium at the back
   C. Meconium coming out of the bowel ostium at the front
   D. Meconium coming out of the bowel ostium caudally

5. **Histopathological examination of the posterior enteric remnant reveals that its walls contain**:

   A. Columnar epithelium
   B. Simple squamous epithelium
   C. Stratified squamous keratinized epithelium
   D. Pseudostratified Columnar epithelium

6. **Dorsal enteric fistulas are classified as**

   A. Cranial defects
   B. Open neural tube defects
   C. Closed neural tube defects
   D. Disorder of notochord formation

7. **The notochord formation begins when the cells in the primitive streak migrate**

   A. Cranially
   B. Caudally
   C. Laterally
   D. Transversely

8. **Split notochord syndrome represents an extremely rare and pleomorphic form of spinal dysraphism characterized by**

   A. A persistent communication between the endoderm and the mesoderm
   B. A persistent communication between the endoderm and the ectoderm
   C. A persistent communication between the ectoderm and mesoderm
   D. A persistent communication between the ectoderm, endoderm, and mesoderm

9. **Which neuroimaging technique can aid in the diagnosis of dorsal enteric fistula**?

   A. Ultrasound
   B. X-ray
   C. CT scan
   D. PET scan

10. **What is the most common location of the dorsal enteric fistula**?
    A. Colon
    B. Distal ileum
    C. Cecum
    D. Duodenum

Answers

1. B
2. D
3. A
4. B
5. A
6. C
7. A
8. B
9. C
10. A

References

1. Lazareff JA. Neural tube defects. Singapore: World Scientific Publishing; 2010.
2. Hoffman CH, Dietrich RB, Pais MJ, Demos DS, Pribram HF. The split notochord syndrome with dorsal enteric fistula. AJNR Am J Neuroradiol. 1993;14(3):622–7.
3. Bentley JF, Smith JR. Developmental posterior enteric remnants and spinal malformations: the split notochord syndrome. Arch Dis Child. 1960;35(179):76–86 [cited 2022 Aug 26]. https://doi org/10.1136/adc.35.179.76.
4. Srivastava P, Gangopadhyay AN, Gupta DK, Sharma SP. Split notochord syndrome associated with dorsal neuroenteric fistula: a rare entity. J Pediatr Neurosci. 2010;5(2):135–7 [cited 2022 Aug 26]. https://doi.org/10.4103/1817-1745.76112.
5. Dhawan V, Kapoor K, Singh B, Kochhar S, Sehgal A, Dada R. Split notochord syndrome: a rare variant. J Pediatr Neurosci. 2017;12(2):177–9 [cited 2022 Aug 26]. https://doi.org/10.4103/jpn.JPN_120_16.
6. Thompson DNP. Gastrulation: current concepts and implications for spinal malformations. J Korean Neurosurg Soc. 2021;64(3):329–39 [cited 2022 Aug 26].
7. Sadler TW. Langman's medical embryology. Lippincott Williams & Wilkins; 2023.

Chapter 10
Neuroenteric Cyst of the Spine

Theogene Uwizeyimana, Sage Ishimwe Marie Consolatrice, and Natnael Shimelash

Test your learning and check your understanding of this book's contents: use the "Springer Nature Flashcards" app to access questions using ▶ https://sn.pub/QCsfpd.
To use the app, please follow the instructions in Chap. 1.

10.1 Introduction

Neurenteric cysts (NEC) are rare congenital abnormalities of the spine that usually happen when there is an abnormal connection between the primitive endoderm and ectoderm [1]. This condition is usually presented in a spectrum of lesions. Kubie and Fulton described these spinal axis lesions made up of heterotopic endodermal tissue in 1928 [1]. The lesions often appear during the third week of human embryonic development, where the neurenteric canal passes through the early notochordal plate and connects the yolk sac and amniotic cavity. This happens when the proper separation of the endoderm and notochord is prevented by the persistence of the ordinarily transitory neurenteric canal, and this connection results in the presence of mucus-secreting epithelium similar to that found in the gastrointestinal system [1, 2]. Since the discovery, the terminology of these lesions has been challenging, with the first term being teratomatous cysts in 1928, intestinomas in 1934, and neurenteric cyst in 1954 by Holcomb and Matson. These confusions in naming are usually due to the presentation of lesions in spectrum.

T. Uwizeyimana (✉) · S. I. M. Consolatrice · N. Shimelash
School of Medicine, University of Global Health Equity, Butaro, Rwanda

K. F. AlAli, H. T. Hashim (eds.), *Congenital Spine Malformations*,
https://doi.org/10.1007/978-3-031-59031-3_10

NEC account for 0.7–1.3% of all spinal tumors, with males being more affected than females. The condition affects individuals of all ages from neonates to older people in 70s, however the majority of reported incidence were among children and young adults [1, 3]. NEC target different location of the spine, ranging from intra or extradural to intra or extramedullary, however the majority (78–90%) of cases are found in intradural and extramedullary [3]. In many literatures, these lesions are reported as case reports and case series. In this chapter, we therefore gathered and described NEC from pathogenesis to clinical presentation, diagnosis to clinical management, and prognosis and clinical outcome.

10.2 Pathogenesis

The pathogenesis of NEC arises from early dysembryologic events occurring during the third week of the human embryologic development.

By the end of the second week, the embryoblast is formed, resulting in the production of the epiblast and hypoblast layers of the bilaminar disc. By the third week following fertilization, the Gastrulation phase commences and resulting in the formation of the trilaminar germ layer. This phase ensues the apoptotic grooving, proliferation, and then migration of epiblast cells (later called ectodermal cells) to form the trilaminar germ layer which includes the ectoderm, mesoderm, and endoderm. The ectoderm later develops in to the Skin and Central nervous system, mesoderm into vital organs such as kidneys, liver, and muscles and endoderm in to mainly the gastrointestinal lining and to some extent respiratory lining.

Ectoderm cells subsequently migrate through the primitive pit towards the precordial plate to form the notochord canal that runs between the endoderm and ectoderm. In the following days the notochord canal continues its dissent and intercalates into the embryonic endoderm. The intercalated floor of the canal undergoes apoptosis opening the floor of the canal. This results in the creation of a semicircular notochordal plate opening to the yolk sac and the Primitive Neurenteric Canal (PNC) connecting the Amniotic cavity (above the ectoderm) with the yolk sac. The notochordal plate continues to morph by approximating its edges to form a canal which then internally proliferates to close the lumen of the PNC and form the notochord. The notochord then detaches and elevates from the endoderm.

NECs are formed due to abnormal detachment and/or elevation of the notochord from its endodermal base. However, there is no consensus on the exact pathogenesis of NECs. Literature identifies five possible mechanisms for the formation of NECs.

10.3 The PNC Lumen Fails to Close

The notochord is separated by endodermal cells forming a diverticular projection of endodermal tissue.

The notochord adheres to the endodermal tissue failing to detach.

The notochord fails to elevate after detachment.

Abnormal notochord development secondary to incomplete ectoderm-endoderm separation.

All mechanisms result in intradural, extramedullary growth of endodermal cells within the central nervous system. This shows in the peculiar histopathology of NECs, as they are lined by non-ciliated, simple, pseudostratified, and columnar or cuboidal epithelium with characteristic proteinaceous secretions.

10.4 Clinical Presentation of Neuroenteric Cyst (NEC) of the Spine

The clinical manifestation of NEC can be subtle and is dependent on the cyst's location on the spine [4]. NEC are most often incidentally detected on imaging in the early 20s and 30 years of age [5]. These cysts can be found anywhere within the body, including the brain, mediastinum, abdomen, pelvis, and even under the skin. Symptomatic NECs are characterized by size-dependent myelopathic and/or radicular symptoms [3].

They are more abundant in the cervical and thoracic regions and are uncommon in the craniovertebral junction, lumbar, and sacral regions [6, 7]. The majority of these cysts are found in the ventral spinal cord's intradural and extramedullary compartments, with less than 5% found in the intramedullary compartment [3]. Symptoms in the cervical region may include progressive neck pain, pain in both shoulders that is unresponsive to medical treatment, and no history of trauma. A neurologic examination may reveal the normal or abnormal motor function and sensation in the upper limbs, which does not rule out the diagnosis but rather necessitates further investigation [8].

NECs can affect the thoracic region of the spine, causing progressive midback pain, midthoracic intercostal pain, upper extremity weakness, prickling sensation, and motor deficits. Trunk stretching frequently aggravates thoracic back pain and sleeping in the opisthotonos position relieves it. Furthermore, NEC rarely affect the lumbar and sacral vertebrae, and when they do, a patient may experience urinary and fecal incontinence, pain at the affected site that can migrate to the lower extremities and cause problems with motor function in the lower half of the body, localized spinal pain, numbness and altered sensations, impotence, and lower limb weakness [9].

NECs of the brain may cause headache progressively increasing in intensity, dizziness, memory impairment, gradual onset swallowing difficulties (dysphagia) and hearing noises in the ears (tinnitus) [10]. In almost half of the cases, NECs are associated with bony abnormalities of the spine and are linked to different conditions such as spina bifida, split cord malformation among others [6]. Further to disrupting the normal shape of the bone of the spine, NECs can be linked with gastrointestinal malformations, anal atresia and renal malformations. Aside from the more common signs and symptoms, the pediatric population has witnessed a wide range of other clinical manifestations including meningeal signs, impairment of the lower motor function, long-lasting fevers [4].

10.5 Diagnosis of Neuroenteric Cyst (NEC) of the Spine

Given that NEC is a disease that comes on slowly and does not have obvious symptoms at first, the history taking, and physical examination would be insufficient to diagnose it [1]. A full history and physical examination, on the other hand, always guide the investigation and management plans. Therefore, thorough investigations are required to avoid missing this life-threatening condition. For NECs, diagnostic imaging and histopathology are performed in additional to history taking and physical examination.

10.5.1 Diagnostic Imaging

Diagnosis using imaging especially Computerized Tomography (CT) and Magnetic Resonance Imaging (MRI) are the standard investigations used to diagnose neurenteric cysts. MRI, however, has proven to be superior to CT in delineating the cyst shape and its link to anatomical parts around it. Hence, MRI is considered as the gold standard for the diagnosis of NECs [1, 3].

10.5.2 Diagnostic Histopathology

A group of mucin-producing simple columnar or cuboidal ciliated and nonciliated goblet cells surrounding a central cyst cavity has been identified as the classic histopathological diagnosis of NECs [1, 3]. Intramedullary cysts stain positively for glial fibrillary acidic protein, whereas extramedullary cysts typically stain negatively. On the surface, neurenteric cysts are made up of a thick superficial layer that envelopes a straw-colored fluid collection. Fluid composition variations include "milky," "blackish," and "clear jelly" appearances. The mucus-secreting columnar epithelium that lines the wall of the neurenteric cyst is identical to the respiratory or gastrointestinal epithelium [1].

10.6 Management of Neuroenteric Cysts (NECs) of the Spine

Surgical removal is the first-line management of NECs. Total excision of the lesion is the best intervention when considering recurrence [2]. However, the ventral inclination of NECs and the proximity of the lesions to the spinal cord may impede total excision. In such cases, partial resection, cyst fenestration, and simple aspiration have been used as alternate methods [11].

Posterior, anterior and lateral surgical approaches have been used to resect NECs, with variable success rates. Although there is no agreement on the top surgical approach, the posterior approach was found to be the most utilized method in NEC resection. This approach is limited by the ventral position of most NECs, which may lead to the spinal cord covering the lesion when approached posteriorly. However, cord manipulation and cyst aspiration are proven techniques to improve access. The posterior approach offers less intraoperative difficulty leading to fewer complications. Potential intra-operative complications with the posterior approach include spinal cord, dural, and/or nerve root injury [2]. The need for frequent aspiration during this approach increases the risk of spillage that may lead to chemical meningitis. In addition, difficulty to control muscle and epidural venous bleeding may lead to hematomas.

The second most utilized approach in NEC resection is the anterior method. This approach provides a more adequate plane of access to NECs that are ventrally located and does not require frequent aspiration of the cyst thus reduces risk of leakage. However, it has a higher surgical difficulty increasing the risk of neurovascular accidents, fusion failures, cerebrospinal fluid leaks, and hematomas.

The least often used method for resecting NECs is the lateral approach. However, it is most suitable to resect lateral and anterior cranio-cervical lesions. It allows a cranio-caudal view and access to the cyst-cord margin and allows access with the least manipulation of the local anatomy, thus has a good cosmetic outcome for neck incisions [2]. This technique has comparable risk as the anterior and posterior approaches.

10.7 Prognosis and Clinical Outcomes

Once total resection is performed, the prognosis of NECs is good. However, surgical morbidity that includes symptoms worsening and failure to return to pre-disease state have been identified in 11% and 18% of cases respectively. The postsurgical recurrence of cysts is another reported scenario, and it was found to range from 0% to 37% of reported cases [1]. According to the literature, recurrence rates are higher in patients who had partial resection than those who underwent total resection [12]. However, the rarity of the illness and limited long-term follow-up studies make it hard to truly estimate the recurrence. Usually, NEC presents as a benign tumor, however, if not treated well it can lead to neurological deficits and/or grow into a malignant tumor [13].

10.8 Conclusion

NECs are rare congenital spine abnormalities that manifest symptomatically in the second decade of life. The clinical manifestation of NEC can be mild, depending on where the cyst is located on the spine. In order to properly diagnose this illness, diagnostic imaging and histology are used in addition to a detailed history taking and physical examination. The prognosis for NECs is good after complete resection. However, those who underwent partial resection experienced postsurgical recurrence.

Multiple Choice Questions

1. **The most common locations of the neurenteric cysts of the spine are**:

   A. Cervical and lumbar regions
   B. Thoracic and lumbar regions
   C. Cervical and thoracic regions
   D. Lumbar and sacral regions

   Answer: C

2. **Which of the following statement about the neurenteric cyst of the spine is correct**:

   A. Neurenteric cysts are most often incidentally detected on imaging in the early 20s and 30 years of age
   B. Neurenteric cysts of the spine are very common and easily detectable on spinal X-ray
   C. Neurenteric cysts of the spine are rare medical conditions but the history taking, and full physical examination are enough to diagnose them when located on the spine
   D. Neurenteric cysts of the spine cannot be congenital, but it is a life-threatening condition

   Answer: A

3. **Which one of the following imaging modalities is used to diagnose neurenteric cyst of the spine and has been proven to best delineate the cyst shape and its relation to the surrounding anatomical structures**:

   A. Computerized Tomography (CT) scan
   B. Magnetic Resonance Imaging (MRI)
   C. X-rays
   D. Ultrasound

   Answer: B

4. **Histopathology is one of the diagnostic tests of neurenteric cysts of the spine. Which among the following statements about the histopathological finding of the neurenteric cyst of the spine is correct**?

   A. A group of mucin-producing simple columnar or connective tissues has been identified as the typical histological diagnostic of neurenteric cysts
   B. The classic histopathological diagnosis of neurenteric cysts has been identified as a group of stratified squamous epithelium or cuboidal ciliated and nonciliated goblet cells surrounding a central cyst cavity

C. The classic histopathological diagnosis of neurenteric cysts has been identified as a group of mucin-producing simple columnar or loose connective tissue
D. The classic histopathological diagnosis of neurenteric cysts has been identified as a group of mucin-producing simple columnar or cuboidal ciliated and nonciliated goblet cells surrounding a central cyst cavity

Answer: D

5. **The pathogenesis of neurenetric cysts culminates in**:

A. Intradural, extramedullary growth of endodermal cells within the central nervous system
B. intradural, extramedullary growth of mesodermal cells within the central nervous system
C. intradural, extramedullary growth of neural cells within the gut
D. None of the above

Answer: A

6. **Which of the following is true about the surgical approach to NECs**

A. The lateral approach is the most utilized approach to surgically remove NEC
B. Aspiration of NECs is the ideal management approach to NEC
C. The posterior approach is the most utilized approach to surgically remove NEC
D. Lateral approach is suitable to resect lateral and posterior lesions craniocervical lesions

Answer: C

7. **Which approach allows the best vantage for the cord-cyst margin**?

A. Posterior approach
B. Lateral approach
C. Anterior approach
D. Antero-lateral approach

Answer: A

8. **Which of the following is not true about NEC formation**?

A. It is formed when the PNC lumen fails to close
B. It is formed when the notochord is separated by endodermal cells forming a diverticular projection of endodermal tissue
C. It is formed when the notochord fails to elevate after detachment
D. All are true

Answer: D

References

1. Savage JJ, Casey JN, McNeill IT, Sherman JH. Neurenteric cysts of the spine. J Craniovertebr Junction Spine. 2010;1(1):58 [cited 2022 Oct 30]. Available from: https://www.jcvjs.com/article.asp?issn=0974-8237;year=2010;volume=1;issue=1;spage=58;epage=63;aulast=Savage;type=0.
2. Garg N, Sampath S, Yasha TC, Chandramouli BA, Devi BI, Kovoor JME. Is total excision of spinal neurenteric cysts possible? Br J Neurosurg. 2008;22(2):241–51.
3. Baek WK, Lachkar S, Iwanaga J, Oskouian RJ, Loukas M, Oakes WJ, et al. Comprehensive review of spinal neurenteric cysts with a focus on histopathological findings. Cureus. 2018;10(9):e3379 [cited 2022 Oct 30]. Available from: https://www.cureus.com/articles/14161-comprehensive-review-of-spinal-neurenteric-cysts-with-a-focus-on-histopathological-findings.
4. Rauzzino MJ, Tubbs RS, Alexander E, Grabb PA, Oakes WJ. Spinal neurenteric cysts and their relation to more common aspects of occult spinal dysraphism. Neurosurg Focus. 2001;10(1):e2.
5. Bhatt AS, Mhatre R, Nadeesh BN, Mahadevan A, Yasha TC, Santosh V. Nonneoplastic cystic lesions of the central nervous system-histomorphological spectrum: a study of 538 cases. J Neurosci Rural Pract. 2019;10(3):494–501.
6. Lan ZG, Richard SA, Lei C, Huang S. Thoracolumbar spinal neurenteric cyst with tethered cord syndrome and extreme cervical lordosis in a child: a case report and literature review. Medicine (Baltimore). 2018;97(16):e0489.
7. Gopakumar S, Gadgil N, McDonald MF, Gadot R, Ropper AE. Neurenteric cyst: case report and operative video. Cureus. 2020;12(6):e8714 [cited 2022 Dec 7]. Available from: https://www.ncbi.nlm.nih.gov/pmc/articles/PMC7372244/.
8. Al-Ahmed IH, Boughamoura M, Dirks P, Kulkarni AV, Rutka JT, Drake JM. Neurosurgical management of neurenteric cysts in children. J Neurosurg Pediatr. 2013;11(5):511–7.
9. Liu SC, Feng YC, Lin CC, Chiou YH, Weng KP. Upper spinal neurenteric cyst presenting as right upper abdominal pain and sudden onset of lower limb paralysis: a case report. Pediatr Neonatol. 2020;61(4):453–4 [cited 2022 Dec 7]. Available from: https://www.pediatr-neonatol.com/article/S1875-9572(20)30019-X/fulltext#relatedArticles.
10. Gavrjushin AV, Chelushkin DM. Intra-axial neurenteric cyst of medulla: case report and literature review. Cureus. 2021;13(5):e15361 [cited 2022 Dec 7]. Available from: https://www.ncbi.nlm.nih.gov/pmc/articles/PMC8245625/.
11. Salehani A, Howell S, Harmon D. Management of a cervical spine neurenteric cyst via an anterior surgical approach: illustrative case. J Neurosurg Case Lessons. 2021;1(5):CASE20119 [cited 2022 Dec 7]. Available from: https://www.ncbi.nlm.nih.gov/pmc/articles/PMC9241353/.
12. Yang T, Wu L, Fang J, Yang C, Deng X, Xu Y. Clinical presentation and surgical outcomes of intramedullary neurenteric cysts. J Neurosurg Spine. 2015;23(1):99–110 [cited 2022 Dec 7]. Available from: https://thejns.org/spine/view/journals/j-neurosurg-spine/23/1/article-p99.xml.
13. Chavda SV, Davies AM, Cassar-Pullicino VN. Enterogenous cysts of the central nervous system: a report of eight cases. Clin Radiol. 1985;36(3):245–51 [cited 2022 Dec 7]. Available from: https://www.sciencedirect.com/science/article/pii/S0009926085800489.

Chapter 11
Dermal Sinus

Naseem Wajdi, Nael Wajdi, and Yasir Khaleel Hameed

> Test your learning and check your understanding of this book's contents: use the "Springer Nature Flashcards" app to access questions using ▶ https://sn.pub/QCsfpd.
> To use the app, please follow the instructions in Chap. 1.

11.1 Introduction

Dermal sinus is a rare congenital malformation that falls under the category of occult spinal dysraphism. It occurs when cutaneous ectoderm and neuroectoderm incompletely separate at focal area between the third and fifth week of gestation presenting later as dermal indentation remnant of incomplete neural tube closure [1]. The extent of incomplete separation determines how deep the tract can penetrate, potentially reaching subcutaneous, fascia, dura, or even intracranial neural tissue [2].

The reported occurrence of dermal sinus is roughly 1 out of 2500 live births, with locations reported all the way along the midline neuraxis and distributed as lumbar (40%), sacral (23%), sacrococcygeal junction (13%), lumbosacral (12%), thoracic (10%), and cervical (<1%) [3, 4]. The incidence of dermal sinus is not limited to a specific gender or linked to certain genetics. Dermal sinuses are typically found above the intergluteal crease [2].

N. Wajdi (✉) · N. Wajdi · Y. K. Hameed
College of Medicine, University of Baghdad, Baghdad, Iraq

K. F. AlAli, H. T. Hashim (eds.), *Congenital Spine Malformations*,
https://doi.org/10.1007/978-3-031-59031-3_11

In the past, the initial presentation of a dermal sinus was as a CNS infection causing a swift decrease in neurological function due to inflammation or pressure. But now, they are more frequently detected by general practitioners during physical exams [5].

Dermal sinus tracts are linked to inclusion tumors like dermoids, epidermoids, and teratomas. They are also linked with tethered cord affecting less than 1% of those with this condition [1].

11.2 Embryogenesis

The neural tube is formed by the neuroepithelial layer, which is an infold of the ectoderm. Neural tube closure begins between the 15th and 17th day after conception (after gastrulation). The structural abnormality arises during growth from the failure to fully separate the ectoderm and neural ectoderm, creating a skin fistula that connects the spinal cord and subcutaneous layers [5].

In the case of dermal sinus tract, there are two theories to explain the pathology.

The first one being that, during embryonic development, the neural ectoderm folds and separates from the ectoderm in a process known as dysjunction [2]. This is crucial for mesoderm insertion, which is the origin of both the musculature and the vertebral column, thereby separating the spinal cord from the overlying skin [6]. If this process is flawed, a stalk remains that connects the skin's ectoderm to the underlying neuroectoderm [7].

Another explanation for the formation of dermal sinuses could be a flaw in the formation of the notochord, leading to a sagittal split in the spinal cord and the persistence of a connection between the cutaneous, endoderm, and mesenchymal tissue [2].

The lining of the formed tract is mainly desquamated-substance secreting epithelial cells, explaining the associated formation of dermoid and epidermoid tumors.

When the connection is opened to the skin from one side and into the dura on the other side, it is called a complete sinus. A complete sinus opens to the skin through a hole and into the dura on the ventral side. Sometimes, the tract could be partially closed at one side creating a partial connection [7].

11.3 Clinical Presentation

Most dermal sinuses are diagnosed in patients under the age of 5, <10% in 6–10 years, and only a few in older than 20 [8].

Patients present in a wide range of presentations with most cases being asymptomatic. However, they may present with infection, neurological compromise, urinary symptoms, and foot deformities [4].

Upon examination, patients usually have cutaneous manifestations as a midline skin dimple, mostly at the lumbar region. It could be accompanied by other skin manifestations such as pigmentation changes, raised plaques, tufts of hair, telangiectasias, and skin tags [8]. Rarely, some patients may have spinal lipoma and human tail [9].

It is important to be highly cautious when it comes to dimples located above the intergluteal fold, regardless of imaging results. If an infant experiences meningitis caused by rare organisms, any dimple found in the midline should be closely scrutinized [10].

A CSF leak may also be present, indicating a connection between the thecal sac and the skin [11]. Being open to the external environment carries the risk of infection providing direct access to the sac leading to signs of erythema, induration, pus formation and discharge [10]. Thus, a suspicious, recurrent, and unexplained infection at the site should prompt a thorough and detailed search for a sinus through physical examination and imaging. The infection may also extend deeper and result in a diffuse infection (meningitis) or form a focus of infection locally (abscess), which could be intramedullary, subdural, or epidural [10].

Neurological manifestation is a feature of older children and may include deterioration secondary to cord tethering to the tract or compression from a tumor [2]. Symptoms may include weakness, changes in sensation, reflexes, gait, decreased muscle tone in the sphincters, or problems with bowel or bladder control. These are usually a result of a compression from a tumor or tethering to the tract [6]. Hence, even though dermal sinus tracts are a rare cause of tethered cords, it's crucial to examine patients with such tracts for the presence of a tethered cord [1].

If deterioration is more gradual, the presentation may be as gait problems, pain, scoliosis, motor or sensory deficits, or orthopedic deformities resembling other forms of occult spinal dysraphism (Fig. 11.1).

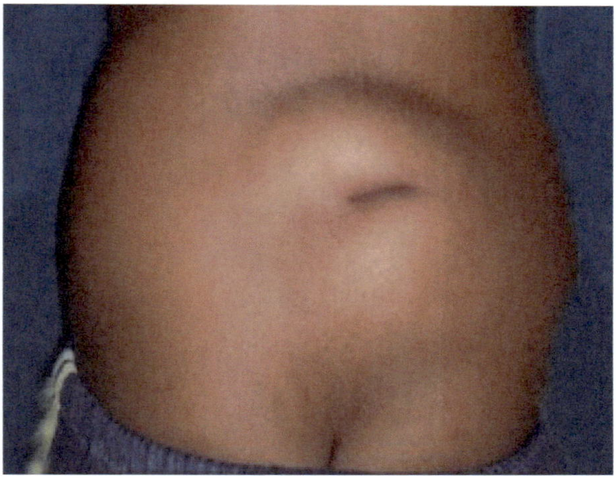

Fig. 11.1 Dermal sinus tract seen at lumbar vertebral level [12]

11.4 Diagnostic Studies

It is important to first undergo a radiological evaluation before attempting to surgically explore or remove dermal sinuses. Attempts to insert a probe or inject contrast materials should be avoided as they can result in infections or damage to deep tissue while not providing diagnostic value [2].

Magnetic Resonance Imaging (MRI), with or without contrast, is the modality investigation of choice for patients with suspected dermal sinus. It can detect the tract itself on T2 weighted imaging as well as associated pathologies that may concur such as other types of spinal dysraphisms, intraspinal extension, syrinx, inclusion tumors, and spinal abscesses [7]. T1-weighted or proton density images are used when the tract path within the spinal cord may be difficult see due to layers of fat.

When assessing for meningitis, lumbar puncture should be done above the documented dermal sinus tract by a few levels (Fig. 11.2).

A CT scan of the brain can be used to check for other conditions, such as ventriculitis, brain abscess, and hydrocephalus. Urinary tests such as urodynamic evaluation can also be done to assess the patient's urinary function, especially in those who have no neurological symptoms [7].

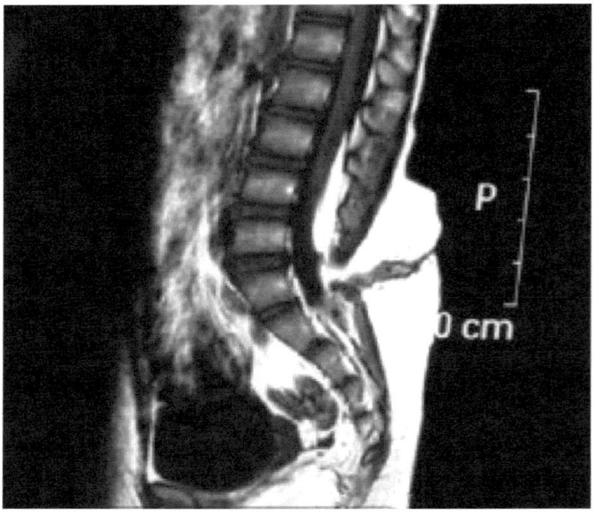

Fig. 11.2 Tethered cord and lipomyelomeningocele seen on T1 weighted MRI scan. This is because of the stalk that extended to the intradural space [12]

11.5 Management

Conservative treatment is contraindicated. Thus, surgical intervention can be done either to treat a secondary neurological deterioration due to infection, as a treatment for a complication such as a tethered cord, or as a prophylaxis in healthy patients [2]. For patients with severe neurological problems, surgical intervention should be done prophylactically to slow the progression of neurological decline [10].

In case of meningitis, immediate antibiotic therapy should be commenced according to local resistance charts.

As for the surgery itself, it is done under general anesthesia and the patient is positioned face-down with appropriate steps taken to avoid pressure points. IONM is always used to monitor the patient.

An incision is made around the lesion and, using methylene blue solution, the sinus tract is emphasized. Then, the tract is then carefully dissected through the fascial, muscular, and bony layers reaching the dura, which is then explored. The part of the tract within the spine along with any associated dermoid tumors is removed with caution to avoid spilling content into the body. If there is an intraspinal abscess, it is drained and a thorough spinal wash is performed.

The area should also be explored thoroughly for the presence of a tethered filum to be excised while monitoring the patient's neurological status. The presence of a tight filum may be underestimated on MRI, so it is important to actively search for it. To prevent recurrence, the entire sinus tract must be removed [7]. Advances in microneurosurgical methods have made full or nearly full removal of cysts achievable in recent cases [13].

In 30% of patients, the tract was discovered to terminate on the dural surface, in 18% it ended in an intraspinal tumor, and in 12% it terminated in the conus. Arachnoiditis was present in 33% of patients, and intraspinal abscess was identified in 25% [7].

Any dermal sinuses located above the sacrococcygeal locale must be surgically examined, regardless of imaging results. This is because no imaging method can accurately reveal the details within the spine [4].

Earlier suspicious, diagnosis, and surgical intervention are of importance because they allow for a better outcome and less complications in the future when compared to patients presenting late as an infection or tumor progression. Any delay in the diagnosis gives time to neurological deficits to develop and this results in a more difficult operation [6].

Even if the MRI results are normal and the passage is located above the crease in the buttock area, it is still advised to undergo surgical exploration, as the passage may be overlooked if it is not in the right angle for the imaging [6].

11.6 Complications

Complications may include wound infection, dehiscence, CSF leak, deteriorating neurological function, and recurrence of inclusion tumors [10]. If a wound breakdown occurs, repairing it can be challenging. The presence of skin vascular anomalies may hinder skin healing [7].

Hydrocephalus can be treated with the addition of a VP shunt or ETV In instances of ventriculitis, it is wise to place a temporary drain while waiting for antibiotics to take effect, both intrathecally and intravenously [7].

11.7 Follow Up

Follow up and monitoring should be done with regular clinical exams, urodynamic testing, and MRI scans in case of a concern of an intraspinal abscess spreading upward [7].

Follow up by imaging is required to check for complications and residual dermoid tissue left which may end in recurrence of inclusion tumors [10].

Subtotal resection is most commonly associated with recurrences, while total excision leads to rare recurrences. If they do occur, they necessitate another surgical intervention for removal. Therefore, it is recommended to have regular check-ups with contrast MRI in the first postoperative year. For patients who have undergone multiple unsuccessful surgeries or have significant fibrosis, radiation therapy may provide relief [13].

11.8 Outcome

The better the condition at the time of the operation, the better the outcome, with most cases having an excellent outcome, especially neurologically intact patients [2]. Those who were neurologically intact will typically remain as such, and those who already have a deficit will improve or stabilize [10].

Multiple Choice Questions

1. ***Dermal sinus is a subtype of which spinal dyspharism***:
    - Apperta
    - **Occulta**
    - Cystica
    - None of the above
2. ***Dermal sinus is most likely to occur in***:
    - Cervical region
    - Thoracic region

- Lumbar region
- Sacral region
- **Lumbosacral region**

3. ***Dermal sinus is most likely to be formed during embryonic life***:

- At the first week of gestation
- Between first and third weeks of gestation
- **Between third and fifth weeks of gestation**
- Between sixth and eighth weeks of gestation
- After the eighth week of gestation

4. ***The modality of choice in the diagnosis of dermal sinus is***:

- X-ray
- US scan
- CT scan
- **MRI scan**

5. ***Patients with dermal sinus are usually presented as which of the following***:

- Infection (meningitis, abscess)
- CSF leak
- **Cutaneous manifestation (skin dimple)**
- Neurological manifestation (weakness, gait)
- Orthopedic deformity

6. ***Which of the following regarding dermal sinus epidemiology is true***:

- It is more common in males
- It is linked with a specific gene mutation
- The incidence is 1:1000 per live births
- **The incidence is 1:2500 per live births**
- It is commonly found below the intergluteal crease

7. ***Which of the following methods results in a WORSE outcome***:

- Operating prophylactically on a patient with limb weakness
- Marking the lesion with methylene blue solution
- Imaging a child with frequent atypical meningitis
- **Presence of vascular anomalies on the skin**
- Usage of IONM during surgery

8. ***The following is strongly associated with a higher risk of recurrence***:

- Excision of the tract with dural exploration
- Total resection of the tract
- **Subtotal resection of the tract**
- Follow up with MRI scan post operatively
- Searching actively for a tight filum seen on MRI

9. ***Regarding the management of dermal sinus***
    - It is usually done for cosmetic reasons
    - Cannot be done prophylactically to prevent complications
    - Antibiotics should not be given before surgery is done
    - Conservative treatment is recommended in most cases
    - **A normal MRI scan does not avoid the need for surgery**
10. ***Which of the following patients is expected to have a better prognosis***
    - A 6-year-old male patient presented as meningitis
    - **A 3-months-old female patient with a skin dimple**
    - A 10-year-old female presented with foot deformity
    - A 1-year-old male presented with CSF leak
    - A 2-year-old female with a red, tender mass on the back

References

1. Ackerman LL, Menezes AH, Follett KA. Cervical and thoracic dermal sinus tracts. A case series and review of the literature. Pediatr Neurosurg. 2002;3:137–47.
2. Roth J, Beni-Adani L, Xiao B, Sira LB, Constantini S. Spinal dermal sinuses. In: The spina bifida. Springer; 2008. p. 515–24.
3. McIntosh R, Merritt KK, Richards MR, et al. The incidence of congenital malformations: a study of 5964 pregnancies. Pediatrics. 1954;14:505–22.
4. Radmanesh F, Nejat F, El Khashab M. Dermal sinus tract of the spine. Childs Nerv Syst. 2010;26(3):349–57.
5. Bevan R, Leach P. Infected congenital cervical dermal sinuses leading to spinal cord abscess: two case reports and a review of the literature. Childs Nerv Syst. 2020;37(1):225–8.
6. Ackerman LL, Menezes AH. Spinal congenital dermal sinuses: a 30-year experience. Pediatrics. 2003;112(3):641–7.
7. Rocco D. Textbook of pediatric neurosurgery. Springer International Publishing; 2020.
8. French BN. Midline fusion defects and defects of formation. In: Youmans J, editor. Neurological surgery. Philadelphia: Saunders Company; 1990. p. 10811235.
9. Samura K, Morioka T, Hashiguchi K, Yoshida F, Miyagi Y, Yoshiura T, et al. Coexistence of a human tail and congenital dermal sinus associated with lumbosacral lipoma. Childs Nerv Syst. 2008;25(1):137–41.
10. Wright ZG, Rozzelle CJ. Dermal sinus tracts. In: Occult spinal dysraphism. Springer; 2019. p. 165–73.
11. Papaevangelou G, Tsitsopoulos PP, Flaris N, Iliadis C, Tsonidis C. Dermal sinus tract of the thoracic spine presenting with intramedullary abscess and cranial nerve deficits. Pediatr Neurosurg. 2015;50(6):339–43.
12. Singh I, Rohilla S, Kumar P, Sharma S. Spinal dorsal dermal sinus tract: an experience of 21 cases. Surg Neurol Int. 2015;6(18):429.
13. Gupta SK, Singh P, Gupta RK, Sharma R, Nehete LS. Infected congenital lumbosacral dermal sinus tract with CONUS epidermoid abscess: a rare entity. Childs Nerv Syst. 2020;37(3):741–7.

Chapter 12
Split Cord Malformations

Sarah Zuhair Kurdi

Test your learning and check your understanding of this book's contents: use the "Springer Nature Flashcards" app to access questions using ▶ https://sn.pub/QCsfpd.
To use the app, please follow the instructions in Chap. 1

12.1 Introduction

Split cord malformations are rare and complex occult spinal dysraphism and one of causes for tethered cord syndrome, in which any part of spinal cord is divided into two symmetrical or non-symmetrical parts by a dorsal or ventral septa [1–3].

Although SCM can occur alone, may associated with other spinal and nonspinal anomalies (e.g., lipoma, kyphoscoliosis, hemivertebra, hypoplastic vertebra, meningomyelocele and dermoid cyst) [4].

There are two types of SCM but not all malformations fit these types and this classification provides a framework for surgical intervention.

1. Type I split cord malformation (formerly diastematomyelia) in which osteocartilaginous septum divided the spinal canal in sagittal plane and spinal cord into two parts surrounded by separated thecal sacs.
2. Type II split cord malformation (formerly diplomyelia) is characterized by midline fibrous septum which extend from the dura and separate spinal cord into two parts within single thecal sac and spinal canal [5].

S. Z. Kurdi (✉)
Kufa University-College of Medicine, Al-Sader Medical City, Najaf, Iraq

K. F. AlAli, H. T. Hashim (eds.), *Congenital Spine Malformations*,
https://doi.org/10.1007/978-3-031-59031-3_12

12.2 History

SCMs first described in the seventeenth century. Historically, in Greek the terms diastematomyelia "cleft medulla" and diplomyelia "double medulla" were used to characterize these anomalies which in 1992 grouped as split cord malformations by Pang and his colleagues [5].

12.3 Embryology

The theory that most commonly used to describe embryogenesis of SCMs was originally described by Bremer and then modified by Pang and his colleagues as a Unified theory of embryogenesis [6, 7].

The basic error occurred during gastrulation in which midline integration of notochord failed, so that the adhesion between endoderm and ectoderm persist by the two unfused heminotochords that causes an **accessory neurenteric canal** (ANC) formation around which an endomesenchymal tract (EMT) condensed and divided the heminotochord into two hemineural plates [8].

The persistence of the anterior end of ANC will cause malformations of intestinal tract while the posterior end leads to cutaneous malformations like dermal sinus, angiomas, dermoid, hypertrichosis, whereas the intermediate **part** result in a split in the neural placode and the notochord.

Around day 28, meninx primitiva cells appeared between the neural plate and the notochord become involved within endomesenchymal tract. The fate of these cells is important in the classification of SCM by forming dura and bone.

If primitive meninx cells (meninx primitiva) incorporated into endomesenchymal tract, double dural tubes will formed around the hemicords and due to their osteogenic potential a median bony spur will form and separate the dural sacs that is SCM type I. This bony spur usually anteroposterior attached to the posterior vertebral body. Rarely, it attached dorsally to the spinous process.

The spur divided the spinal canal either symmetrically or asymmetrically into two parts. Harwood-Nash et al. described asymmetry in 50% of cases, in which one of the hemicords can be hypoplastic [9].

The osteogenic effect of the meninx cells on the developing neural arches explain the hypertrophic fusion of adjacent laminae at the level of split cord [10].

In the majority of type I split cord malformation, the septum is located in the lumbar area and less frequently lower thoracic, cervical and upper thoracic regions in decreasing order of frequency. Occasionally, two levels separated septa occurred . The splitting of the cord can extend over several segments then reunite into normal cord.

In contrast, in type II Split cord malformation, meninx primitiva cells are excluded from the endomesenchymal tract and a fibrous septum will form from the mesenchyme separating the hemicords [11]. So the double cords will lie within a single thecal sac and single spinal canal. Always this septum is adherent to the medial aspect of the hemicords with firmly attached to the ventral and/or dorsal wall of dura so fibrous septum like bony septum is a real tethering lesion.

The **timing** may be the reason behind why some EMT entrap meninx cells, whereas other are not . Since the endomesenchymal tract formation occurred around day 18 to 22 of gastrulation in a rostrocaudal direction, a **rostral tract** would complete its development before meninx cells appearance, whereas a **caudal tract** will entrap meninx cells during its development so that proximal split in cervical and high thoracic SCMs are almost exclusively type II, whereas type I located in the lumbar and lower thoracic regions [12, 13].

Rarely, dorsal EMT persist lead to dermal sinus tract derived from ectodermal cells. In type I SCM, it extend from the skin through myofascial layers and neural arches to the bone spur so the dermal sinus tract is **extradural** and does not account for the tethering while in type II, it is attached to the hemicords, and may lead to dermoid cyst formation which will cause compression of the spinal cord [14].

25% of SCMs usually associated with open neural tube defects that may result in a full blown myelomeningocele or hemimyelomeningocele [15, 16].

12.4 Clinical Features

Patients with SCM may be asymptomatic with only cutaneous marks. The clinical signs and symptoms most likely arise from traction of the spinal cord against the medium septum which prohibit the ascent of the cord within the thecal sac. It usually presented at 6 years, neurologic signs and symptoms that become more evident at time of walking.

In general, clinical presentations can be divided into: (1) cutaneous abnormalities, (2) pain, and (3) neurological deficits [17] (Table 12.1).

During infancy, cutaneous lesions will bring the parents attention to neurosurgeon which is present in up to 92% of patients which are usually found **caudal** to the level of the split because spinal cord migrated rostrally in relation to the spinal column after the formation of splitting [5].

Most common cutaneous stigma is a patch of hair or hypertrichosis in the thoracic or lumbosacral regions which is highly specific for SCM. This may be coarse and long hair referred to as **faun's tail**. In addition to hemangioma, a dermal sinus, sacral dimple, meningocele, lipoma, or may be associated with the spur. Sometimes deformities of feet are present at birth [17–19].

During childhood as the child begins walking and control sphincters, the neurologic deficits usually appear such as weakness and spasticity of lower limbs, an ulcer due to anesthesia, new onset of bowel or bladder incontinence and loss of sensation in the sacral dermatomes which are due to spinal cord tethering.

Table 12.1 Clinical features of SCM

PAIN	Low backache Shooting pain down the leg
CUTANEOUS ABNORMALITIES	Faun's tail or hypertrichosis Angiomatous malformation Lipoma Dermal sinus or dimple Prominent spinous process Meningocele
NEUROLOGIC ABNORMALITIES	Short leg and hypoplasia of calf and thigh Clubfoot Clawed toes Adducted forefoot Muscle weakness Sensory disturbance Diminished sensation in the leg or perianal area Scoliosis Distended bladder Impotence

SCM split cord malformation

About 50% of patients with SCMS have structural asymmetry of the lower limbs referred to as **neuro-orthopedic syndrome** which is a triad of limb length discrepancy, clubfoot deformity and muscles atrophy. Often the shorter leg is ipsilateral to a smaller hemicord. While about 20% of patients will have structural symmetry with asymmetrical neural deficits which is usually due to hydromyelia of one hemicord [5, 20, 21].

Kyphoscoliosis may also occurred which often progressive due to structural vertebral anomalies like hemivertebrae [17].

In older children and adults, axial back pain is more common and is often localized and more intense at the level of the split. 10% of patients, radicular symptoms may be present which may be due to scoliosis or other bony deformities [5].

Although the clinical presentations are very similar between the two types, there are three exceptions for type 1 SCM which are: (1) more likely have dysesthetic pain in the legs (2) scoliosis is more common; and (3) signs of chronic sympathetic denervation are more common such as thin hairless skin, unhealed ulcer, anhydrosis [12].

Surgeon evaluating a patient with SCM should keep in mind associated abnormalities that may require additional surgeries such as scoliosis, myelomeningocele, tethered cord secondary to terminal lipoma or thickened filum, Chiari II malformation and syrinx [5] (Fig. 12.1).

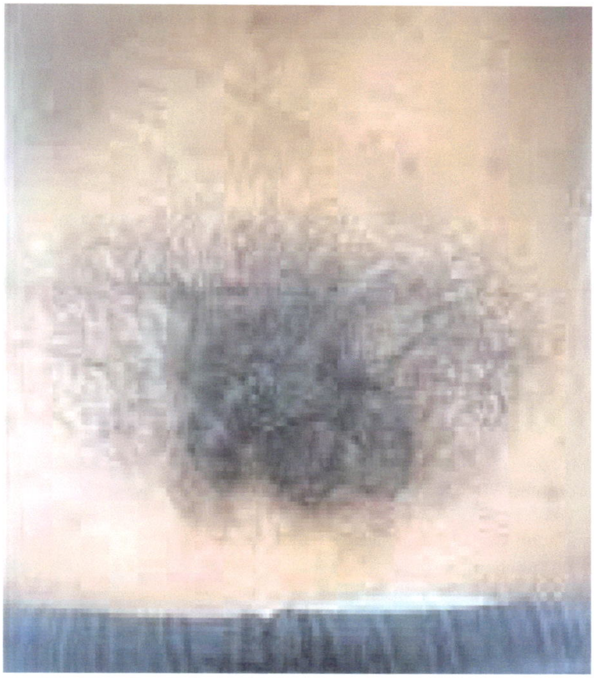

Fig. 12.1 Faun's tail (hypertrichosis) a patch of coarse and long hair in the lumbar region which is highly specific for SCM

12.5 Diagnostic Aids

Magnetic resonance imaging (MRI) is a screening test of choice and its very important for diagnosis and surgical planning. The main feature is the presence of two hemicords which usually reunited after two to three vertebral segments. T2-MRI can distinguish the presence of one or two subarachnoid spaces, type I SCM have an "owl sign" as in Fig. 12.2 and in type II hypointense fibrous band may appeared (Fig. 12.3). Also syrinx may appear proximal to the split and extend into one or both hemicords [5].

Computed tomography (CT) best visualize the bony spur of type I SCM. Also associated bony anomalies which occurred in more than 85% of patients which include bifid vertebrae, butterfly vertebrae, bifid laminae, Klippel-Feil syndrome, hemivertebrae and scoliosis.

Hypertrophic arch are often fused to the laminae of adjacent segments which known as intersegmental laminar fusion. Intersegmental laminar fusion with spina bifida are pathognomonic for type I SCM [5, 11, 17].

Overall, both CT and MRI imaging are important for diagnosis of SCM and the entire spinal column should be imaged.

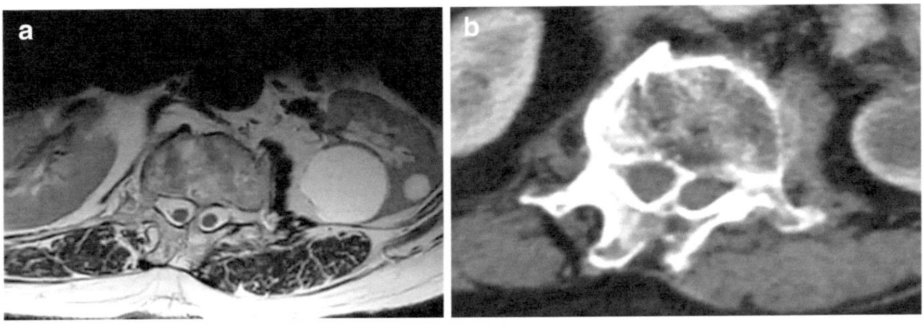

Fig. 12.2 (**a**) T2 axial MRI at level of L1 showing owl sign of type I SCM with two hemicords contained within two separated thecal sacs. (**b**) Axial CT scan bone window at L1 lumbar vertebra showing bony septum that separate completely the spinal canal with bifid spinous process

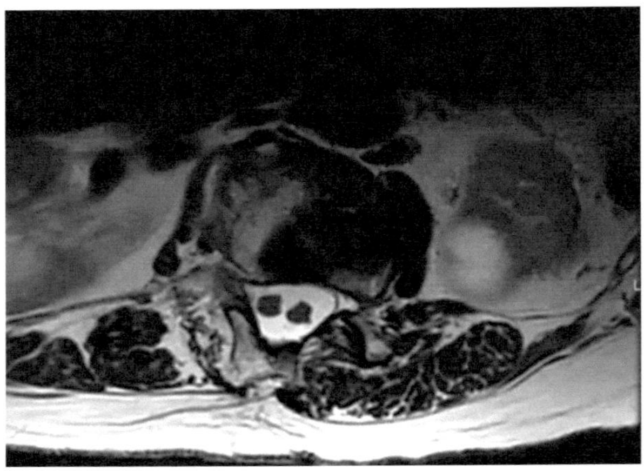

Fig. 12.3 Axial T2 weighted MRI at level of T10 of Type II SCM showing single thecal sac with two hemicords, the fibrous septum is not clear in this image in such case CT Myelography is more sensitive

CT myelography is superior to MRI in identification and localization of the fibrous septum and myelomeningocele manqué but it is unnecessary unless ambiguity after MRI happened [5].

Plain radiographs may be helpful for the diagnosis of scoliotic deformities, long-term follow-up as well as setting a marker for incision.

Urodynamic studies (preoperative and postoperative) are important as in one study reported incidence of abnormal urodynamic studies up to a 75% of patients, despite lack of symptoms [17, 18].

12.6 Management

Both types of SCM are a cause of spinal cord tethering. Any patient with symptoms or signs attributed to this malformation should be operated in order to relieve symptoms, preserve function and possibly reverse neurological deficits.

In children the mere presence of split cord is an indication for prophylactic surgery due to risk of neurologic deterioration. In both types of SCM, the aim of surgery is removing the septa and all other tethering bands [10].

In the newborns, surgery should be delayed for about 3 months so they can tolerate anesthesia and will have well developed soft tissues and meninges, allowing good surgical closure with better outcome.

In asymptomatic adults there is less convincing evidence to support prophylactic surgery, and most adult surgery have been done for symptoms and/or progressive neurological deficits. However, worsening of the neurological function can occurred after trauma or strenuous exercise. Therefore, surgery is recommended in asymptomatic adults who are healthy and have physically vigorous life, while old or infirm adults and those with sedentary lifestyle managed conservatively.

The management required team work of pediatrics, physical therapy, pediatric neurosurgery, pediatric urology and orthopedics.

12.7 Operative Technique for Type I SCM

Under general anesthesia the patient positioned prone as for a laminectomy.

Surgery is often performed with intraoperative neuromonitoring which strongly considered in all cases of SCM, including continuous SSEP, MEP, EMG and anal sphincter monitoring. Intraoperative C arm or fluoroscope can be useful in localization of the level of lesion [5].

Surgery started by making a standard midline skin incision above and below the level of SCM localized by radiograph that correlated with the preoperative MRI then lumbosacral fascia incise and subperiosteal dissection of the paraspinous muscles is done. The monopolar cautery should be used with caution in dissecting muscles, because area of missing bone must be expected.

Then spinous processes of laminae above and below the lesion are removed using a rongeur. With partial laminectomy at the caudal aspect of the lamina above and the rostral aspect of the lamina below.

The ligamentum flavum, incised vertically and cottonoid patty is used for protection of the dura then it removed by a small Kerrison punch.

The median septum is always extradural and can be either purely bony or partly cartilaginous but purely cartilaginous septa are rare. The medial walls of the double dural tubes forming a sleeve for the bone in the sagittal plane. Over the area of septum, a small rongeur or high-speed drill or angled Kerrison punch is used to perform bilateral paramedian laminectomies, while the midline lamina and spinous process preserved to prevent avulsion of bony septum prematurely as it is often fused with the undersurface of the lamina and the base of the spinous process. With a Penfield dissector, the septum is felt from above and below and the palpable segment of spur removed using a rongeur, and complete dissection of bony spur from dura down to the level of the dorsal surface vertebral body which removed using high-speed diamond drill. Embedded in the septum is central artery that can cause profuse bleeding if avulsed [5, 17, 22].

Then midline dural opening is done starting at normal level above extending down elliptically on sides of the spur and then down in the midline and this dural sleeve or pouch is excised (Fig. 12.4). Any remaining bony spur must be trimmed down to avoid retethering [5].

Inspect medial aspect of both hemicords, with removal of blood vessels and fibrous bands which often adherent to the dural sleeve tightly, between hemicords and median dural sleeve there may be **Paramedian dorsal nerve roots** which are nonfunctional and should be cut before resection of the dural sleeve then any associated lesion (fatty filum, sinus tract, or lipoma) should also be resected [3]. Most neurosurgeons prefer division of a normal filum terminale in patients with a low-lying conus either from same incision or second one [5].

After that watertight closure of the dorsal dura is performed, fibrin glue can be used if needed. The Closure of the ventral dural defect is not required and undesirable because of adhesions that will form between the dura and the posterior longitudinal and these suture lines can potentially tether the hemicords [23].

A drain is inserted in subfascial plane and closure of soft tissues in anatomical layers is performed. Postoperatively, the patient should lie flat in bed for 1–2 days to prevent CSF leak.

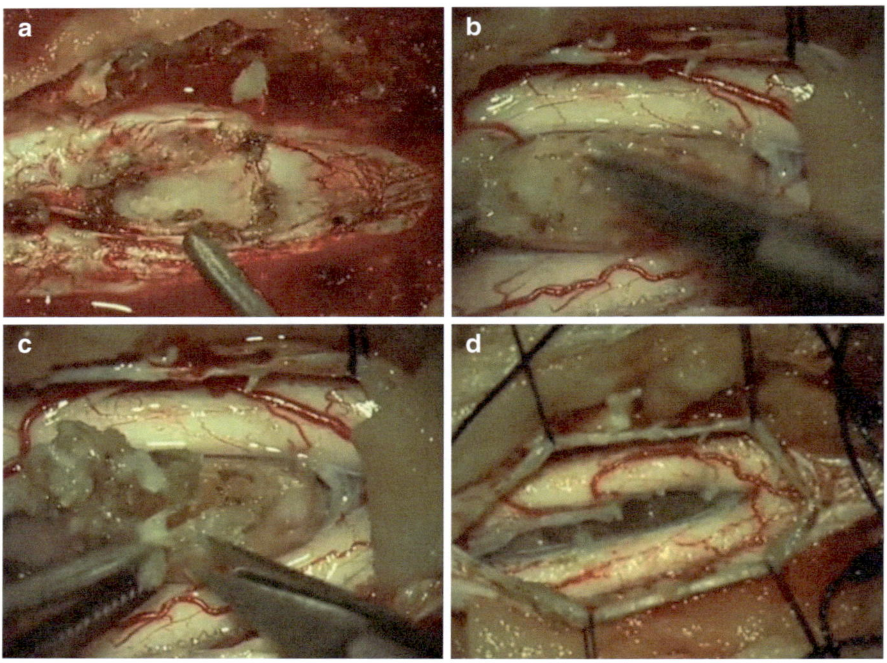

Fig. 12.4 Type I SCM operative views. (**a**) Double thecal sacs with median bony septum. (**b**) Identification of anterior dural wall after removal of bony septum. (**c**) Resection of anterior dural wall. (**d**) Final view of two hemicords after total removal of bony septum and anterior dura before reconstruction into single dural sac

Prone position is preferred by some neurosurgeons to prevent adhesion of the spinal cord to the dural suture line [5]. Standard prophylaxis against deep venous thrombosis should be undertaken for adolescents and adults. The Foley catheter is removed once mobilization start, with monitoring of post voiding residual urine.

12.8 Operative Technique for Type II SCM

In type II, a fibrous septum is found intradurally between the double cords in midline. Three patterns of such septa are encountered (1) complete fibrous septum: the least common stretched between the ventral and dorsal dura. (2) Purely ventral fibrous septum: Slightly more common stretched between ventral dura and ventromedial aspects of the hemicords. (3) Purely dorsal septum: the most prevalent kind that attaches the dorsal dura to the dorsomedial aspects of the hemicords.

Surgery is done under general anesthesia with neurophysiological monitoring and skin incision extend one level above and below the site of split then lumbosacral fascia incised and paraspinal muscles reflected. Fused and Hypertrophic laminae which are common in type I SCMs, are rarely seen in type II so laminectomy for these lesion is easy and safe [24]. Then midline dural opening is done and a septum is exposed (Fig. 12.5). Intracleft exploration is not recommended as all fibrous septa are thin and the length of the split is short so the hemicords will apposed close to each other.

Like the bony septa, the fibrous septa are also found near the distal end of the split. The point of attachment between septum and hemicords is proximal to the attachment point between the fibrous septum and dura due to the fact that the septum was moved upward during rostral migration of the spinal cord.

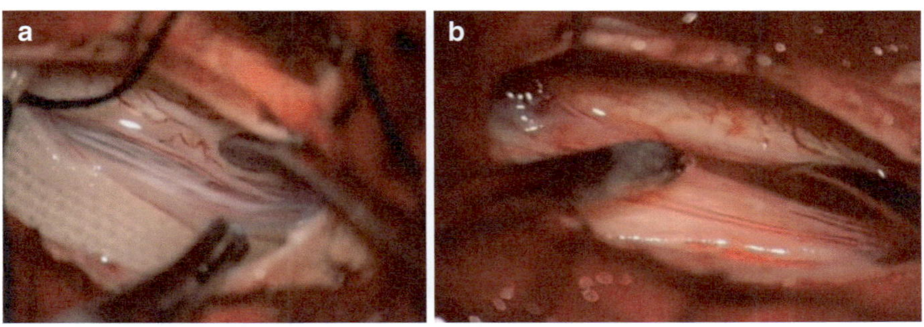

Fig. 12.5 Type II SCM operative views. (**a**) Fibrous septum is seen separating the two cords. (**b**) The two cords after resection the septum

Then fibrous septum is cut and any other tethering lesions such as paramedian dorsal nerve roots and myelomeningocele manqués which are common in type II SCMs also cut. Filum terminale dethered in the same way. Dorsal dural incision sutured watertight and closure of the rest of anatomical layers is done.

12.8.1 Complications

Cerebrospinal Fluid Leakage especially in previously treated open neural tube defect due to poor myofascial coverage which should be managed by bed rest in lateral or prone position for 3 to 5 days and oversewn the suture line that leak, if persist lumbar drain may be used. If not responding exploration with primary repair of dura or use of fascia lata or dural substitute with fibrin glue or DuraGen if needed.

Epidural or subdural hematoma presented with delayed neurological deficits and need urgent MRI for diagnosis, meticulous hemostasis and use of drain for 24 h may decrease their incidence.

Infection including meningitis, epidural or subdural empyema can occurred which can be avoided by perioperative antibiotic and early treatment of CSF leak.

Transient urinary retention is not uncommon which can last few days to several months and is more common in adults with type I SCM than in children which can be managed by folly catheter or intermittent catheterization. Permanent bladder dysfunction occurs in less than 3% of patients and evaluated by urodynamic study [25].

Neurological injury can caused by contusion, traction, or direct injury by surgical instrument or a drilling and that observed more with type I SCM which can be prevented by careful manipulation of the spinal cord [17].

Symptoms recurrence may be due to retethering (although regrowth of the septal spur is very rare but it has been reported), sometimes adhesion by scar tissue at the surgical site, or undiagnosed secondary lesion. The diagnosis is made on clinical grounds. MRI will demonstrates enlargement or new syringomyelia with low lying conus or the presence of secondary tethering elements [5, 26].

12.9 Outcome

In more than 90% of patients, Surgery will results either in improvement or stabilization of neurological deficits [27]. Axial back pain will show improvement in the majority of cases, Progressive motor and sensory deficits show the most pronounced improvement while bladder function will regained in only one third of patients [5].

Most favorable Outcomes observed in prophylactic repair of asymptomatic patients with only cutaneous stigmata [19]. So earlier surgery is associated with better long-term outcome.

7% of patients develop new sensorimotor deficits which are transient in the majority however, 3% of new permanent deficits have been observed [21, 27].

Multiple Choice Questions

1. **Type I SCM is characterized by**
   (a) Double spinal canal
   (b) Hemivertebra
   (c) Bony septum
   (d) Tethered cord
   (e) All of above
2. **Type II SCM is characterized by**
   (a) Double dural sac
   (b) Bony septum
   (c) Open neural tube defect
   (d) More common in thoracic region
   (e) Cured by dethering of filum terminale
3. **All of the following regarding embryology of SCM are true except**
   (a) Persistence of posterior end of accessory neurenteric canal
   (b) The basic error occurred during gastrulation
   (c) Incorporation of meninx cells contribute to bony septum formation
   (d) 25% of SCMs associated with open neural tube defect
   (e) Pang unified theory is the most common theory explain this malformation
4. **Cutaneous stigma which is highly specific for SCM is**
   (a) Dermal sinus
   (b) Hypertrichosis
   (c) Sacral dimple
   (d) Lipoma
   (e) Capillary hemangioma
5. **Asymmetric neural deficits may be due to**
   (a) Long medium septum
   (b) Presence of lipoma
   (c) Tethering of one hemicord
   (d) Hydromyelia of one hemicord
   (e) Scoliosis

6. **36 years old male with SCM, which of the following is the common symptoms**
   (a) Urinary incontinence
   (b) Dysesthesia
   (c) Lower limb weakness
   (d) Axial back pain
   (e) Club foot
7. **5 years old boy presented by his mother to the neurosurgeon, she was worried about his awkward gait and frequent fall during running for the last 3 months after examination the doctor found abnormal hair on his back with bilateral spastic weakness of the lower limbs and sent for MRI and diagnosed him with SCM type 1, which of the following is incorrect?**
   (a) MRI show an owl sign.
   (b) Weakness result from mass effect of bony septum on the spinal cord.
   (c) Hypertrichosis is the most important sign for localization of the pathology.
   (d) The doctor arranged patient for surgical intervention.
   (e) The doctor need to order urodynamic study.
8. **8 years old female with new urinary incontinence for 1 month diagnosed as type II SCM, which of the following is correct?**
   (a) The two hemicords with double thecal sac separated by fibrous septum.
   (b) More common in female.
   (c) More common in the cervical area.
   (d) Surgery can be delayed after puberty.
   (e) CT myelography is superior to MRI in diagnosis of the fibrous septum.
9. **Regarding management of SCM which of the following is incorrect**
   (a) Only type I need surgical intervention
   (b) The aim of surgery is removing the median septum and all other bands.
   (c) Asymptomatic young healthy adults with SCM there is no need for surgery.
   (d) The mere presence of SCM is an indication for prophylactic surgery in children.
   (e) Both (a) and (c)
10. **CSF leak in patient with operated SCM occur due to?**
   (a) Unsutured anterior dural defect
   (b) Previously treated meningocele with SCM
   (c) Hydrocephalus
   (d) Dermal sinus
   (e) All of the above

Answers and Explanation

1. (e) All of the above, Type I SCM is characterized by bony septum that split the cord and spinal canal into two parts, the clinical presentation is due to spinal cord tethering. Associated vertebral anomalies like hemivertebra can occur.
2. (d) More common in thoracic region, Type II SCM is characterized by medium fibrous septum with splitting of the cord into single thecal sac, management of this condition required removal of fibrous septum and any dural bands or associated lesion with cutting of filum. SCM per se are closed NTD.
3. (a) Persistence of posterior end of accessory neurenteric canal, accessory neurenteric canal in its anterior end if persist lead to intestinal malformation while posterior end cause dermal sinus tract and the intermediate part are responsible for SCM.
4. (b) Hypertrichosis, a hair patch is observed in the thoracic or lumbosacral regions which is highly specific for SCM. This hair may appear long and coarse named as faun's tail.
5. (d) Hydromyelia of one hemicord, about 20% of patients have an asymmetric neural deficit which is usually associated with hydromyelia of one hemicord.
6. (d) Axial back pain, in adult with undiagnosed SCM, Axial back pain is common and may be the only symptom and is localized and more intense at the level of the split. A radicular symptoms may be present in 10% of cases which may be due to simple scoliosis or to the bony deformity.
7. (b) Weakness result from mass effect of bony septum on the spinal cord. MRI will show an owl sign characteristic of type I SCM with two hemicords and the usual presentation in this age group will be spastic weakness of lower limbs, ulcers due to anesthesia and bowel or bladder incontinence which are due to tethered cord by bony septum and he need urgent surgical intervention.
8. (e) CT myelography is superior to MRI in diagnosis of the fibrous septum. In type II SCM the two hemicords present within single sac separated by fibrous septum, there is no sex preference and its more common in the lumbar region. The presence of SCM is an indication for prophylactic surgery and any neural deficit will be an urgent surgical condition to preserve neural function.
9. (e) Both (a) and (c), surgery is recommended in asymptomatic adults with SCM who are healthy and have physically vigorous life, both types of SCM are tethering lesions and required surgical intervention prophylactically in children due to risk of neurological deterioration.
10. (b) Previously treated meningocele with SCM, cerebrospinal Fluid Leakage occurred more with previously operated open neural tube defect due to poor myofascial coverage and multiple dural adhesion.

References

1. Borkar SA, Mahapatra AK. Split cord malformations: a two years' experience at AIIMS. Asian J Neurosurg. 2012;7(2):56–60. https://doi.org/10.4103/1793-5482.98643. PMID: 22870152; PMCID: PMC3410161
2. Venkatramana NK, Spinal dysraphic states, Ramamurthi and Tandon's textbook of neurosurgery, vol 1, 3rd edition , Jaypee Brothers Medical Publishers ,2012, p (287).
3. Schijman E. Split spinal cord malformations: report of 22 cases and review of the literature. Childs Nerv Syst. 2003;19(2):96–103.
4. Alnefaie N, Alharbi A, Alamer OB, Khairy I, Khairy S, Saeed MA, Azzubi M. Split cord malformation: presentation, management, and surgical outcome. World Neurosurg. 2020;
5. Raskin JS, Litvack ZN, Selden NR. Split spinal cord, Youmans and Winn neurological surgery. 7th ed. Philadelphia: Elsevier; 2017. p. 3322–30.
6. Bremer JL. Dorsal interstitial fistula, accessory neurenteric canal, diastematomyelia. Arch Pathol Lab Med. 1952;54:132.
7. Pang D, Dias MS, Ahab-Barmada M. Split cord malformation I. A unified theory of embryogenesis for double spinal cord malformations. Neurosurgery. 1992;31:451–81.
8. Conley AM, Ward JD. Occult spinal dysraphism and the tethered spinal cord, Benzel's spine surgery, vol. 1. fourth ed. Elsevier; 2017. p. 1713–7.
9. Harwood-Nash DC, McHugh K. Diastematomyelia in 172 children: the impact of modern neuroradiology. Pediatr Neurosurg. 1991;16:247–51.
10. Mitchell JB, Pang D. Surgical management of spinal dysraphism, Schmidek and sweet operative neurosurgical techniques, vol. 2. 6th ed. Elsevier; 2012. p. 899–911.
11. Erşahin Y, Demirtaş E, Mutluer S, Tosun AR, Saydam S. Split cord malformations: report of three unusual cases. Pediatr Neurosurg. 1996;24:155–9.
12. Pang D. Split cord malformation: part II: clinical syndrome. Neurosurgery. 1992;31(3):481–500.
13. Pang D, Acosta F Jr, Gupta N. Spinal dysraphism, pediatric neurosurgery. 1st ed. Landes Bioscience: Georgetoen, Texas U.S.A; 2006. p. 293–305.
14. Saraga-Babić M, Stefanović V, Wartiovaara J, Lehtonen E. Spinal cord-notochord relationship in normal human embryos and in a human embryo with double spinal cord. Acta Neuropathol. 1993;86(5):509–14.
15. Iskandar BJ, McLaughlin C, Oakes WJ. Split cord malformations in myelomeningocele patients. Br J Neurosurg. 2000;14(3):200–3.
16. Pang D, Hou YJ, Wong ST. Chapter 106–1 Classification of spinal dysraphic malformations according to embryogenesis: gastrulation defects and Split cord malformation. Springer Science and Business Media LLC; 2017.
17. Tye GW, Ward JD, Myseros JS. Occult spinal dysraphism and the tethered spinal cord. Elsevier BV; 2005.
18. Proctor MR, Bauer SB, Scott RM. The effect of surgery for split spinal cord malformation on neurologic and urologic function. Pediatr Neurosurg. 2000;32(1):13–9.
19. Sinha S, Agarwal D, Mahapatra AK. Split cord malformations: an experience of 203 cases. Childs Nerv Syst. 2006;22(1):3–7.
20. Warder DE. Tethered cord syndrome and occult spinal dysraphism. Neurosurg Focus. 2001;10(1):1–9.
21. Ozturk E, Sonmez G, Mutlu H, et al. Split-cord malformation and accompanying anomalies. J Neuroradiol. 2008;35(3):150–6.
22. Shivapathasundram G, Stoodley MA. Use of a synthetic dural substitute to prevent ventral retethering in the management of diaste-matomyelia. J Clin Neurosci. 2012;19(4):578–81.
23. The spina bifida. Springer Science and Business Media LLC; 2008.

24. CHAPTER 12. Protocol for management of split cord malformations. Georg Thieme Verlag KG; 2021.
25. Pang D, Zovickian JG, Oviedo A. Long-term outcome of total and near total resection of spinal cord lipomas and radical reconstruction of neural placode. Part II: outcome analysis and preoperative profiling. Neurosurgery. 2010;66(2):253–73.
26. Agarwal A, Kumar A, Shaharyar A. A new radiological sign for split cord malformation type I: "the owl sign". Spine J. 2014;14(9):2271–2.
27. Mahapatra AK, Gupta DK. Split cord malformations: a clinical study of 254 patients and a proposal for a new clinical-imaging classification. J Neurosurg. 2005;103(suppl):531–6.

Chapter 13
Caudal Regression Syndrome

Ahmed Hassan A. Rady, Mohamed Osama Farouk, and Mohammedbaqer Ali Al-Ghuraibawi

Test your learning and check your understanding of this book's contents: use the "Springer Nature Flashcards" app to access questions using ▶ https://sn.pub/QCsfpd.
To use the app, please follow the instructions in Chap. 1

13.1 Introduction

Caudal regression syndrome (CRS) is a rare congenital disease during the antenatal period that is characterized by abnormal development of the spinal cord which leads to poor growth of the caudal half of the body. This disease is also associated with many congenital anomalies such as urologic, gastrointestinal, cardiac, nervous, and orthopedic abnormalities [1, 2].

13.2 Epidemiology

The prevalence of the disease among infants born from non-diabetic mothers is 1–3 per 100,000 live births, while, this number is greatly increased among births from a diabetic mother, around a 150-fold increase. This disease is also referred to as

A. H. A. Rady (✉) · M. O. Farouk
Faculty of Medicine, Ain Shams University, Cairo, Egypt

M. A. Al-Ghuraibawi
Faculty of Medicine, University of Warith Al-Anbiyaa, Karbala, Iraq

K. F. AlAli, H. T. Hashim (eds.), *Congenital Spine Malformations*,
https://doi.org/10.1007/978-3-031-59031-3_13

caudal dysplasia, congenital sacral agenesis, and Sacro-coccygeal dysgenesis. Critical cases of CRS may die so early diagnosis is crucial [3].

13.3 Etiology

The caudal mesoderm mis-develops during the first month of pregnancy, but the exact method by which this sickness manifests itself is still not fully known. Some risk factors have been connected to it. The most crucial factor is whether the mother had diabetes. Additionally, the mother's use of alcohol, cocaine, trimethoprim-sulfamethoxazole, and minoxidil has been linked to certain occurrences. Other possible explanations include the vascular steal theory, fetal hypoxemia, retinoic acid imbalance, and infections. Additionally, genetic changes in the HLXB9, CYP26A1, and HOXD13 gene sequences appear to be more significant in the progression of the illness [4].

13.4 Related Conditions

The Currarino triad or sequence is similar but different than CRS it includes anorectal atresia, coccygeal and partial sacral agenesis, and a pre-sacral mass as a lipoma or a dermoid cyst. Sirenomelia, also known as mermaid syndrome, is characterized by a single midline Lower limb and atypical abdominal umbilical artery. Some doctors describe sirenomelia as the most severe form of CRS (called CRS type V), however, there is some controversy over whether it is a separate disease or not [5].

13.5 Types of CRS and Sirenomelia

There are five types of CRS and seven types of Sirenomelia. CRS was categorized by Pang and Renshaw, while sirenomelia was classified by Pang, Kjaer, Stocker and Heifetz.

- Type I - has complete or partial unilateral sacral agenesis.
- Type II - has varying lumbar and complete sacral agenesis where the ilia articulate with the edges of the lowest vertebrae.
- Type III - has varying lumbar and complete sacral agenesis and the bottom end plate of the lowest vertebrae rests above fused ilia.
- Type IV - soft tissues in both lower limbs are joined together.
- Type V - sirenomelia, has bones of the lower limb combined together.

On the other hand, ***the classification of Sirenomelia***

- Type I - of sirenomelia has the correct number of femurs, tibia and fibula;
- Type II - has one fibula.
- Type III - has no fibulae.

- Type IV - has a femur fused and fibulae fused.
- Type V - has no fibulae and partly fused femurs.
- Type VI - has one femur and one tibia.
- Type VII - has one femur and no tibiae [6–8].

13.6 Signs and Symptoms

Caudal regression syndrome symptoms and severity vary widely from person to person. Most likely, the term "causal regression syndrome" refers to a variety of illnesses; from those with little symptoms to those with severe impairment or potentially fatal sequelae. There are abnormalities that affect the sacrum and lumbar spine. The sacrum may disappear completely. Sacral dysplasia is often associated with narrowing of the lower back, underdeveloped gluteal muscles (hypoplasic hips), dimples in the skin of the lower back (sacral dimples), and flattening of the buttocks [5].

There may also be an abnormality in the lumbar spine. Some patients experience damage or injury to the lower part of the spinal cord, which can lead to various neurological disorders such as: Bladder and bowel control problems, frequent urination, inability to completely empty the bladder (neurogenic bladder) cause anomalies. Urological abnormalities that may be associated with caudal regression syndrome can be significant [9].

Affected infants may also have reduced muscle mass in the legs, clubfoot, or webbed knees (popliteal ptergyium). Some patients with caudal regression syndrome have meningocele, and have a variety of additional ailments, including renal anomalies, upper spine anomalies, facial anomalies such as cleft lip and palate, and conditions in which a thin sheath blocks the anal opening or passageway. May indicate physical findings. The lowest junction of the large intestine (rectum), including the anus, does not develop. This is known as anal atresia or imperforate anus. Congenital heart disease and respiratory complications may also be associated with caudal regression syndrome.

13.7 Diagnosis

Diagnosis of caudal regression syndrome can be made before birth (prenatal), usually by ultrasound of the fetus. Fetal ultrasound can detect some of the defects associated with caudal regression syndrome. Additional tests may be required to detect or assess physical findings that may be related to the disorder. For example, echocardiography is usually done to assess the degree of involvement of the heart. An echocardiogram is a test that uses sound waves to take pictures of the heart. Magnetic resonance imaging (MRI) can also be done to determine the extent of certain abnormalities, such as: Spine defect to evaluate. MRI uses a magnetic field and radio waves to create cross-sectional images of specific organs and body tissues [10].

13.8 Treatment

Treatment may require a coordinated effort by a team of specialists. Pediatricians, neurosurgeons, neurologists, urologists, orthopedic surgeons, orthopedic surgeons, cardiologists, and nephrologists to tailor the treatment of caudal regression syndrome to the specific symptoms experienced by each individual. It also varies from infant to infant based on a variety of factors. Affected infants may require complex medical and surgical interventions. Multiple surgeries may be required to treat certain limb deformities associated with various urinary, spinal, and cardiac abnormalities, anal atresia, and caudal regression syndrome. In addition, anticholinergic drugs can be given to treat urinary system problems [6].

13.9 Prevention

Caudal Regression Syndrome can't be prevented because some of the causes are the result of random genetic changes that you can't predict or prevent. Nevertheless, efforts can be done to reduce the risk by working with healthcare provider to manage blood glucose levels in diabetic mothers during pregnancy [7].

Multiple Choice Questions

1. **3 years old came to the pediatric clinic with difficulty in walking, after careful history and examination the patient was diagnosed as a case of caudal regression syndrome. What is the most important risk factor for developing this Disease:**

   (A) Maternal alcohol addiction
   (B) Maternal cocaine consumption
   (C) Maternal high blood glucose
   (D) Infection

2. **CRS is represented as the following except:**

   (A) Scoliosis
   (B) Congenital sacral agenesis
   (C) Sacro-coccygeal dysgenesis
   (D) Caudal dysplasia

3. **The type IV consists of CRS:**

   (A) Total or partial unilateral sacral agenesis
   (B) Lower limb bones joined together
   (C) varying lumbar and complete sacral agenesis where the ilia articulate with the edges of the lowest vertebrae
   (D) soft tissues in both lower limbs are joined together

4. **Which of the following is the most severe form of CRS:**

   (A) Type IV
   (B) Type V
   (C) Type I
   (D) Type II

5. **The abnormal development of the mesoderm occurs within:**

   (A) 1 month
   (B) 6 months
   (C) 8 months
   (D) 4 month

References

1. Sen KK, Patel M. Caudal regression syndrome. Med J Armed Forces India. 2007;63(2):178–9. https://doi.org/10.1016/S0377-1237(07)80071-2. Epub 2011 Jul 21. PMID: 27407981; PMCID: PMC4925436
2. Devesa J, Alonso A, López N, García J, Puell CI, Pablos T, Devesa P. Growth hormone (GH) and rehabilitation promoted distal innervation in a child affected by caudal regression syndrome. Int J Mol Sci. 2017;18(1):230. https://doi.org/10.3390/ijms18010230. PMID: 28124993; PMCID: PMC5297859
3. Boruah DK, Dhingani DD, Achar S, Prakash A, Augustine A, Sanyal S, Gogoi M, Mahanta K. Magnetic resonance imaging analysis of caudal regression syndrome and concomitant anomalies in pediatric patients. J Clin Imaging Sci. 2016;20(6):36. https://doi.org/10.4103/2156-7514.190892. PMID: 27833778; PMCID: PMC5041376
4. Bicakci I, Turgut ST, Turgut B, Icagasioglu A, Egilmez Z, Yumusakhuylu Y. A case of caudal regression syndrome: walking or sitting? Pan Afr Med J. 2014;26(18):92. https://doi.org/10.11604/pamj.2014.18.92.3683. PMID: 25400859; PMCID: PMC4231316
5. Negrete LM, Chung M, Carr SR, Tung GA. In utero diagnosis of caudal regression syndrome. Radiol Case Rep. 2015;10(1):1049. https://doi.org/10.2484/rcr.v10i1.1049. PMID: 27408660; PMCID: PMC4921155
6. Seidahmed MZ, Abdelbasit OB, Alhussein KA, Miqdad AM, Khalil MI, Salih MA. Sirenomelia and severe caudal regression syndrome. Saudi Med J. 2014;35(Suppl 1):S36–43. PMID: 25551110; PMCID: PMC4362094
7. NORD (National Organization for Rare Disorders). Caudal regression syndrome (2019). Available at: https://rarediseases.org/rare-diseases/caudal-regression-syndrome/#:~:text=A%20diagnosis%20of%20caudal%20regression,usually%20during%20a%20fetal%20ultrasound. Accessed 29 Oct 2022.
8. Caudal regression syndrome (sacral agenesis): Symptoms & causes (no date) Cleveland Clinic. Available at: https://my.clevelandclinic.org/health/diseases/23425-caudal-regression-syndrome. Accessed 29 Oct 2022).
9. Kumar Y, Gupta N, Hooda K, Sharma P, Sharma S, Kochar P, Hayashi D. Caudal regression syndrome: a case series of a rare congenital anomaly. Pol J Radiol. 2017;4(82):188–92. https://doi.org/10.12659/PJR.900971. PMID: 28439323; PMCID: PMC5388306
10. Singh SK, Singh RD, Sharma A. Caudal regression syndrome--case report and review of literature. Pediatr Surg Int. 2005;21(7):578–81. https://doi.org/10.1007/s00383-005-1451-4. Epub 2005 Jun 24. PMID: 15977017

Chapter 14
Segmental Spinal Dysgenesis

Zainab A. Alkhuzaie, Yasser F. Almealawy, and Fatimah Dheyaa Kadhim

Test your learning and check your understanding of this book's contents: use the "Springer Nature Flashcards" app to access questions using ▶ https://sn.pub/QCsfpd.
To use the app, please follow the instructions in Chap. 1

14.1 Introduction

Segmental spinal dysgenesis is considered one of the rare types of congenital spinal malformation where there is agenesis or dysgenesis of the spinal cord. This type of congenital malformations is characterized by segments of abnormal vertebrae and underlying spinal cord but with normal vertebrae above and below the anomaly [1]. It belongs to a group of anomalies called spinal dysraphism, which is a term that is used to resemble congenital malformations of the spine and are classified into an open and a closed type.

The open type is characterized by a defect in the cutaneous tissue above the abnormality which makes the underlying structures uncovered. On the other side, the closed type is covered by normal skin.

SSD falls into the closed category and is further classified into two types which will be discussed later.

SSD was first reported by Winter et al. and was called congenital spinal stenosis [2].

It can affect any portion of the spine but it is higher in prevalence in lumbar or thoracolumbar regions [3, 4].

There is no gender preference and associations have been found with maternal diabetes, anoxia and exposure to intrauterine toxins [5, 6].

Z. A. Alkhuzaie (✉) · Y. F. Almealawy · F. D. Kadhim
College of Medicine, University of Kufa, Najaf, Iraq

K. F. AlAli, H. T. Hashim (eds.), *Congenital Spine Malformations*, https://doi.org/10.1007/978-3-031-59031-3_14

14.2 Embryogenesis of SSD

The stages of Gastrulation, primary and secondary neurulation are all essential parts of the normal development of the spine [7].

Gastrulation involves transferring from a two-layered embryo composing of an upper layer of ectoderm and a lower layer of endoderm referred to as "bilaminar disc" into a three-layered embryo which involves the mesoderm in addition to the previous two layers and referred to as "trilaminar disc" [7, 8]. This layer is important for development of spinal structures and this process takes place in the third week.

Primary neurulation occurs when an interaction takes place between the notochord and the ectoderm, the result of this interaction is the formation of the neural tube and the folding of which results in formation of the primary neural tube at 3–4 weeks [7].

Secondary neurulation occurs when caudal cells migrate to form secondary tube at 5–6 weeks [7].

The vertebral development occurs at the same time of the development of the notochordal [9]. Any defect in one of these stages can cause malformations of the spinal cord.

Around the same time, the mesoderm that is around the notochord divides into three regions, from lateral to medial are lateral, intermediate and paraxial mesoderm.

42–44 Somites form from the paraxial mesoderm in a craniocaudal orientation [5].

Some of these somites differentiate into sclerotome which gives rise to vertebrae and skeleton and dermomyotome which gives rise to muscle and dermis.

Any loss of notochord segment affects sclerotome only but doesn't affect dermatome nor myotome. This yields several malformations of the vertebral column and costal anomalies [5].

Not only does the notochord cause the ectoderm to transform into the neural tube, however, it also triggers the development of the vertebral body. As a result, when there is an abnormality in the segmental chorda mesoderm embryological components, it alters the initiation of somite formation which leads to absent cord. This likely results from the relationship that is between every vertebra and a level of the spinal cord. This has an impact on how the spinal cord develops [5].

SSD is related to caudal agenesis [10]. It was believed that the defect in embryological development that leads to SSD was in primary neurulation [3]. But data suggest now that malformations occur in the stage of gastrulation.

Some Authors also believed that SSD could be related to unknown genetic defect with normal notochord formation.

There is communication between yolk sac and amniotic sac. This communication disappears in the third week before beginning of primary neurulation. Therefore, SSD is caused by a disturbance of the notochordal mesodermal during gastrulation that is linked to the positional of the apoptosis of cells with an abnormal axial specification [3].

The degree of notochordal cell depletion is related to the severity of disorder.

Segmental spinal Dysgenesis and CRS, i.e. caudal regression syndrome, in the opinion of authors, present different phenotypes along a single malformation spectrum [3]. That is, if the lesion affected is more distally then it is called caudal regression syndrome and if the segment involved is more proximally then it's referred to as SSD [4].

14.3 Pathogenesis of Classification

SSD consist of two types; type 1 refers to congenital agenesis or dysgenesis of segments of the spinal cord and overlying vertebrae associated with narrowing of the spinal canal and gibbus deformity.

The stage of embryology which is affected in type one is gastrulation [5].

In normal process, Ectodermal cells migrate to the inferior primitive streak and then pass inside to the primitive pit, where they spread between the ectoderm and the endoderm to eventually result in the mesoderm, then reunites in the middle to form the notochord or the chordamesoderm [5].

Dysraphic conditions result from any failure of fusion in a given region or from any independent development.

Type 2 is defined as congenital vertebral defect in which there is absence of multiple vertebrae with sever kyphoscoliosis and damage to the involved nerve roots, that are corresponding to the deformed segments, with narrowing of the spinal cord due to mechanical compression and gibbus deformity. Mechanical compression can cause abnormal somitogenesis that cause secondary cord compression.

Mutation in the pathway of notch signaling (MESP 2, a transcription factor for posterior bHLH, and delta-like 3) can be an etiology of this type [5].

The embryological defect in SSD type 2 occurs during somitogenesis (3–6 weeks) where somite resegmentation and segmentation abnormality cause anomalies of the vertebrae that include transitional, butterfly and block vertebrae.

The difference between type 1 and 2 is that Type 2 affects multiple vertebrae due to defect in somitogenesis unlike type1.

14.4 Clinical Features

Patients with closed spinal dsyraphism require extensive clinical assessment to suspect the presence of such conditions as they can often be entirely occult [10].

Tortori-Donati et al. described SSD as an association of complete absence or dysgenesis of segments of lumbar and/or thoracolumbar regions of the spine with abnormalities of the corresponding spinal cord and nerve roots branching from the same level of the spinal cord [11, 12].

Variety of clinical pictures could present, this depends on the severity and level of anomaly and the presence of accompanied anomalies [13].

The typical sign being a bony protuberance of kyphotic gibbus corresponding to the same level of segmental dysgenesis [10, 14].

The degree of severity of the condition varies from mild stenosis of a part of the spinal cord and the spine giving rise to a focally hypoplastic segment without disconnection of two segments of the spine to a more severe form where there is complete absence of segment of the spine cord and aplastic bony spine resulting in two spinal segments and acute kyphosis [10, 15]. However, The spinal segments distal and proximal to the defected segment are of a normal caliber [4].

Regarding neurological functions, about half of patients present with normal findings with the remaining half presenting with various neurological deficits [2] The degree of these neurological disorders depends on both the severity of spinal cord stenosis and how well the remaining segment of the spinal cord functions [16].

Of these neurological findings, spastic paraparesis and neurogenic bladder, which could be further complicated by UTI, vesicoureteral reflux (VUR), in addition to hydronephrosis, are the most common presentations [6, 11]. It is important to note that some patients initially present neurologically intact at birth, but they are susceptible to neurological deterioration later due to spinal instability [17, 18].

Other deformities that can present are those of the lower limbs and can be in form of hypotrophic lower limbs and equinocavovarus feet [10].

Other anomalies may be accompanied including meningioma, lipoma, congenital heart diseases, lung hypoplasia and imperforate anus [2, 13].

A differential diagnosis of SSD is congenital kyphosis type 1 which can be similar and confusing with SSD. This is different from SSD by the absence of spinal stenosis associated with SSD and generally good neurological function at birth, although it may lead to neurological deficit if left untreated [19].

14.5 Investigations

For early detection of spinal congenital anomalies, prenatal screening provides a good opportunity for diagnosing and determining the risk stratification and helps with arranging the needed management plan. Although magnetic resonance imaging (MRI) of the spine considers the gold standard for SDD screening, it is also associated with several challenges, including its cost and the needed time to be performed along with the fact that it is invasive imaging modality and requires sedation in infants. It is highly dependent on factors affecting resolution, such as vascular flow, patient motion, and physiological motion from CSF pulsation. Therefore, spinal ultrasound is considered the best option for congenital anomalies screening; it is safer, less expensive, not invasive, and can be performed portably with no need for sedation. It is worth mentioning that after the age of bone ossification the US has no useful value, therefore for older pediatrics, MRI is the best imaging modality for the diagnosis of SD [20, 21].

If during routine US screening, any abnormalities were identified, fetal MRI is needed subsequently to confirm a spinal abnormality, followed by postnatal imaging. MRI is recommended not only to further characterize the spine anomaly identified by the ultrasound but also to recognize any associated extracranial and cranial abnormalities that the ultrasound has not adequately evaluated. Because of the small size of the fetus and the unavoidable excessive fetal motion, fetal MRI is typically avoided before 18 weeks of gestation [22, 23].

Postnatally, MRI is well established as the gold standard imaging modality for assessing SSD. CT is helpful in providing optimal delineation of bony defects, whereas 3-D reconstructions can also provide enhanced visualization of the overall deformity along with helping in intervention planning.

The severity of the malformation and its segmental level along the longitudinal embryonic axis influences the picture. Both the severity of the clinical deficit and the severity of the morphologic impairment is associated with residual spinal.

Cord function [11].

The imaging findings of the segmental vertebral anomalies involving the thoracolumbar, lumbar, or lumbosacral spine are characterized by a localized deformity of the spine that may be associated with scoliosis or kyphosis and abnormality of the underlying nerve roots, with a low-lying and thickened configuration .The spinal canal may be thinning or even undetectable, and a thick low-lying cord segment may typical be present caudal to the focal abnormality or even interrupted at the gibbus apex of the kyphotic deformity accompanying by hypoplasia or absence of the cord traversing this region [10, 24].

14.6 Management

The management planning for SSD depends on multiple factors including the type, severity, associated complications, and the patient's age; therefore, approaching each patient individually is required. Patients should receive care in tertiary care settings, ideally from a multidisciplinary spinal dysraphism care team, and options for surgical treatment are taken into account on an individual basis. Generally, rigid spinal immobilization is recommended for 12 to 18 months to allow growth and development before spinal fusion. Surgical decompression cannot treat patients born with neurologic dysfunction. To avoid instability at the dysgenic site, those with progressive deformity should receive initiate treatment with a brace [18].

Surgery is indicated in patients who are failing brace therapy or who have neurological functions that are relatively unaffected below the level of the anomaly and in case where radiological examinations reveal significant cord compression. For a better prognosis of congenital spinal deformities, an early surgical intervention, that aims to establish and maintain spinal stability first and then decompression of the cord is advised to balance spinal growth and avoid the development of rigid deformities and secondary structural curvatures.

Although many types of procedures can be performed as indicated, the most common types are decompression and arthrodesis. The surgery should focus on the associated kyphosis, scoliosis, and subluxation at the involved surgical site to create a solid arthrodesis and stop the development of deformity. However, after surgery, a significant number of patients may experience neurological status deterioration or fail to recover [25]. And although postnatal surgical decompression has been reported to prevent worsening neurologic function, there is currently no available treatment for this condition [2, 26].

The surgeon performing the surgical repair should be aware of associated anomalies because they frequently result in the greatest morbidity, such as neurogenic bladder and renal abnormalities.

Multiple Choice Questions

1. **SSD has a higher prevalence in which region in the spine?**
   (a) cervical region
   (b) coccygeal region
   (c) Sacral region
   (d) Thoracolumbar region

2. **Which statement is true regarding SSD type 1?**
   (a) it occurs due to defect in somatogenesis .
   (b) It affects more than one vertebra
   (c) It occurs due to defect of gastrulation
   (d) One of the etiologies of type 2 is a mutation of the pathway of notch signaling (MESP 2, a transcription factor for posterior bHLH, and delta-like 3)

3. **When spinal dysgenesis affects proximal portions of the spine, it is referred to as**:
   (a) caudal regression syndrome
   (b) Segmental spinal dysgenesis
   (c) Filum lipoma
   (d) Myelocele

4. **Regarding SSD, all followings are true, except**
   (a) 50% of patients present with neurological deficit at birth
   (b) Spinal segments distal and proximal to the defected segment are of normal caliber
   (c) Spastic paraparesis is a rare neurological finding
   (d) Other visceral abnormalities may be associated

5. **What is the best radiological option for congenital spinal defects screening?**
   (a) MRI
   (b) Ultrasound
   (c) CT scan
   (d) 3D reconstruction

6. **What is the best radiological option for diagnosis of segmental spinal dysgenesis?**

(a) MRI
(b) CT scan
(c) Ultrasound
(d) 3D reconstruction

7. **Best time to do a fetal MRI is?**

(a) Before 12 weeks of gestation
(b) After 18 weeks of gestation
(c) Before 18 weeks of gestation
(d) After 12 weeks of gestation

8. **The imaging findings of spinal defects are usually characterized by?**

(a) Generalized deformity of the spine with normal nerve roots
(b) Localized deformity of the spine with normal nerve roots
(c) Generalized deformity of the spine with abnormal distal nerve roots
(d) Localized deformity of the spine with abnormal nerve roots

9. **Management plan for spinal defects:**

(a) is the same for all patients and is usually arranged by a multidisciplinary team?
(b) Depends on multiple factors and could involve surgery as an option
(c) Focus in treating the associated anomalies
(d) Aims to completely cure the disease

10. **In a patient who is under the age of 18 months, management by------- is a good option:**

(a) An early surgical intervention
(b) Decompression and arthrodesis
(c) A brace
(d) Rigid spinal immobilization

11. **Which one of these options is not an indication for surgery:**

(a) Patients under the age of 18 months
(b) When other management alternatives have failed
(c) Patients with significant neurological findings
(d) None of the above

12. **The aim of the surgery is:**

(a) To cure the neurological defects
(b) To stop the development of deformity and create a solid arthrodesis
(c) To manage the associated anomalies
(d) None of the above

Answers

1. **D**

2. **C**
3. **B**
4. **C**
5. **B**
6. **A**
7. **B**
8. **D**
9. **B**
10. **D**
11. **A**

References

1. Rossi A, Martinetti C, Morana G, Severino M, Tortora D. Diagnostic approach to pediatric spine disorders. Magn Reson Imaging Clin N Am. 2016;24:621–44.
2. Kim D, Betz R, Huhn S, Newton P. Surgery of the pediatric spine. Stuttgart: Georg Thieme Verlag; 2008.
3. Mahomed N, Naidoo J. Spinal segmental dysgenesis. SA J Radiol. 2009;13(2):29.
4. Coley B. Caffey's pediatric diagnostic imaging.
5. Chellathurai A, Ayyamperumal B, Thirumaran R, Kathirvelu G, Muthaiyan P, Kannappan S. Segmental spinal dysgenesis–"redefined". Asian Spine J. 2019;13(2):189–97.
6. Naik S, Bhoi S, Panigrahi K. Segmental spinal dysgenesis: a rare congenital spinal malformation. Indian J Radiol Imaging. 2019;29(04):480–1.
7. Rufener S, Ibrahim M, Raybaud C, Parmar H. Congenital spine and spinal cord malformations—pictorial review. Am J Roentgenol. 2010;194(3_supplement):S26–37.
8. Kumar J, Afsal M, Garg A. Imaging spectrum of spinal dysraphism on magnetic resonance: a pictorial review., World J Radiol, vol. 9; 2017. p. 178.
9. Chellathurai A, Kathirvelu G, Mukkada P, Rajendran K, Ramani R. Spinal dysraphisms: a new anatomical–clinicoradiological classification. Indian J Radiol Imaging. 2022;31(04):809–29.
10. Goethem J, Hauwe L, Parizel P. Spinal imaging. Berlin: Springer; 2007.
11. Tortori-Donati P, Fondelli M, Rossi A, Raybaud C, Cama A, Capra V. Segmental spinal dysgenesis: neuroradiologic findings with clinical and embryologic correlation [internet]. Am J Neuroradiol. 1999. [cited 1 October 2022]. Available from: http://www.ajnr.org/content/20/3/445%20:724–7.
12. Tokudome K, Ito S, Kato T, Yanase T, Kawarasaki T, Moritomo Y. Segmental spinal dysgenesis with caudal agenesis in a Holstein calf. J Vet Med Sci. 2017;79(2):277–81.
13. Eltorai I. Rare diseases and syndromes of the spinal cord.
14. Sav A. Pathological anatomy of spina bifida. In: The spina bifida; 2008.
15. Sandhu M, Garg A, Gupta A. AIIMS-MAMC-PGI's comprehensive textbook of diagnostic radiology. 3rd ed.
16. Fratelli N, Rich P, Jeffrey I, Bahmaie A, Thilaganathan B, Papageorghiou A. Prenatal diagnosis of segmental spinal dysgenesis. Prenat Diagn. 2007;27(10):979–81.
17. Faciszewski T, Winter R, Lonstein J, Sane S, Erickson D. Segmental spinal dysgenesis. A disorder different from spinal agenesis. J Bone Joint Surg Am. 1995;77(4):530–7.
18. Hughes L, McCarthy R, Glasier C. Segmental spinal dysgenesis: a report of three cases. J Pediatr Orthop. 1998;18(2):227–32.
19. Herring J. Tachdjian's pediatric orthopaedics. 6th ed.
20. Tawfik N, Ahmed A, El-Shafei T, Habba M. Diagnostic value of spinal ultrasound compared to MRI for diagnosis of spinal anomalies in pediatrics. Egypt J Radiol Nucl Med. 2020;51(1)

21. Aboughalia H, Noda S, Chapman T, Revzin M, Deutsch G, Browd S, Katz D, Moshiri M. Multimodality imaging evaluation of fetal spine anomalies with postnatal correlation. Radiographics. 2021;41(7):2176–92.
22. Weinstein SL, Flynn JM. Pediatric orthopaedics. 7th ed. Lippincott William & Wilkins; 2014. p. 756.
23. Masselli G. MRI of fetal and maternal diseases in pregnancy. 1st ed; 2016.
24. Knafl E, Lall N, Love M, Bui C, Steven A. Segmental spinal dysgenesis. Ochsner J. 2020;20(3):244–7.
25. Remondino R, Tello C, Bersusky E, Francheri Wilson A, Noel M, Galaretto E, et al. Surgical treatment of segmental spinal dysgenesis: a report of 19 cases. Spine Deform. 2020;9(2):539–47.
26. Simon E, Pollock A. Prenatal and postnatal imaging of spinal dysraphism. Semin Roentgenol. 2004;39(2):182–96.

Chapter 15
Intradural Lipoma

Ahmed Elnahhas and Ahmed Talaia

Test your learning and check your understanding of this book's contents: use the "Springer Nature Flashcards" app to access questions using ▶ https://sn.pub/QCsfpd.
To use the app, please follow the instructions in Chap. 1

15.1 Embryology

The exact genesis of spinal lipoma is still unknown, but several theories could explain its origin. The developmental error theory, the most accepted one, states that the underlying mechanism is errors occurring during primary and secondary neurulation [1]. The process of primary neuration starts with the appearance of neural folds and neural grooves. The fusion of neural folds forms a neural tube. The next step is the separation of the neural tissue from the cutaneous ectoderm in a process known as disjunction. Premature disjunction occurs when the separation precedes neural fold fusion as in. As a result, mesenchymal tissue from the para-axial mesoderm invades the enfolding neural tissue. This mesenchymal tissue forms adipocytes giving rise to a spinal lipoma [2]. This premature disjunction could be unilateral producing an eccentric spinal lipoma or bilateral producing midline lipoma. The etiology of developmental error theory is not a true neoplasm but a malformation due to the inclusion of atypical fat cells because of unsuccessful neurulation [3]. All three germ layers Ectoderm, mesoderm, and endoderm could be

A. Elnahhas (✉) · A. Talaia
Faculty of medicine, Tanta University, Tanta, Egypt
e-mail: ahmed.31010526@med.tanta.edu.eg

K. F. AlAli, H. T. Hashim (eds.), *Congenital Spine Malformations*,
https://doi.org/10.1007/978-3-031-59031-3_15

found. Histopathological examination of the lipoma showed in some patients that there can be aberrant skeletal muscles, dermoid cysts, and lymphoid tissue, leading some researchers to think of it as a teratoma [1].

During secondary neurulation, the caudal neuropore closes and fuses with caudal eminence (the tail bud) giving rise to a structure known as the neural cord. A cavity is formed within the neural cord, which is connected to the central canal within the primary neural tube forming a secondary neural tube. The distal portion of this secondary neural tube degenerates forming the filum terminal [4]. Therefore, defects in secondary neurulation result in abnormalities in the caudal region of the spinal cord as conus and filar lipomas.

Primary and secondary neurulation are not separate entities but there is a continuity between the formed primary and secondary neural tubes. The processes happening between them were termed "junctional neurulation". Errors in junctional neurulation were thought to be one of the contributory factors to neural tube defects in the thoracolumbar regions [5] and are associated with the formation of a separate but functional conus medullaris [6].

Another theory is the metaplastic theory postulating that the deposition of fat inside the dura is due to connective tissue metaplasia as there are adipocytes that are normally found in the meninges, but this theory failed to explain why most lipomas are found within the thoracolumbar region and the close association between spinal lipomas and other anomalies like spina bifida [7]. Another theory states that atypical fat cells arise from stem cells that form spinal blood vessels. Mesenchymal cells form the spinal vessels instead of fat cells due to inhibitory signals from the neural crest cells preventing the formation of adipocytes. If there are no inhibitory signals due to defective neural crest cells the mesenchymal stem cells form adipocytes forming a spinal lipoma [8].

15.2 Classification

There are many ways to classify spinal lipomas. Initially, spinal lipomas were surgically categorized according to their location in relation to the spinal cord and the posterior root of spinal nerves into 3 classes, dorsal (attached to the dorsal aspect of conus medullaris), caudal (attached to the caudal aspect of conus medullaris and nerve roots may pass through the lipoma), and transitional spinal lipomas (combination of both dorsal and caudal) [9]. After the wide usage of magnetic resonance imaging, 2 more classes were added: filar lipomas and lipomyelomeningocele [10].

Understanding the underlying embryogenesis for spinal lipomas opened the way for new classification methods. The initial classification, Pang classification depending on the underlying embryology included 3 main classes dorsal, terminal, and transitional spinal lipomas. Both dorsal and transitional lipomas occur due to failed primary neurulation while terminal lipoma occurs due to failed secondary neurulation. Afterward, a new class was added known as chaotic lipoma with its developmental origin occurring at junctional neurulation [11, 12]. The most recent model for classification of spinal lipomas according to the embryological origin, Morota classification, divided spinal lipomas into 4 types [13]. In type 1 the etiology is due to primary neurulation failure. It is the typical form in which the lipoma is on the dorsal surface of the spinal cord. In type 2, there is a failed junctional neurulation. The lipoma is attached to the spinal cord but unlike type 1, conus medullaris is malformed and difficult to be recognized by the MRI which is the key difference between type 1 and 2. Type 2 is associated with other conditions like pathological spina bifida and fascial defects. It Includes the chaotic lipoma previously mentioned in other classification methods. in types 3 and 4, the failure occurs at the beginning and the end of secondary neurulation respectively. In type 3 the caudal end of conus medullaris is unformed and connected to the lipoma, thus it corresponds to the caudal type of earlier classifications. The lipoma could extend through the caudal direction to connect with the subcutaneous fat through the sacral hiatus. Unlike type 2 there is no spina bifida or fascial defects. Type 4 spinal lipoma is the result of ineffective degeneration that occurs at the end of secondary neurulation in the filum terminale. Unlike type 3 the caudal end of conus medullaris is normal on MRI and filum terminale appears as linear string-like masses of lipoma.

15.3 Location

Spinal lipomas are rare lesions and form around 1% of all spinal tumors [14]. Defining the exact extent and location of the spinal lipoma in relation to the cord and the dura is important. The differential diagnosis, clinical picture, prognosis, associated congenital anomalies, and management plan could vary according to the location. Spinal lipomas are mostly associated with dysraphism, a condition where the mass within the cord communicates with subcutaneous lipoma through a defect in the posterior elements of the spine. Lumbosacral lipomas are commonly associated with spinal dysraphism. Lumbosacral lipomas usually as intradural mass with no evidence of spina bifida in 25% of the cases [15]. Non-dysraphic intradural lipomas are usually in the thoracic region followed by the cervical and the cervicodorsal regions. They usually involve several segments in the spinal cord [16]. True intramedullary lipomas are very rare [17]. The position of the lipoma in relation to the cord is usually posterior and located around the midline so they distort and expand the spinal cord.

15.4 Diagnosis

15.4.1 Imaging Modalities

Multiple imaging modalities could be used to visualize intradural lipomas. Table 15.1 shows the key characteristics of intradural lipoma using different imaging modalities. Magnetic resonance imaging is the most sensitive imaging modality for diagnosing spinal lipomas and for planning surgeries. It shows the anatomical relationship between the lipoma and the surrounding structures. It also helps in detecting common associated congenital anomalies including meningoceles and split cord malformations. There is a short T1 relaxation time due to the high proportion of fatty tissue. Thus, on T1 weighted images, spinal lipomas have hyperintense and a clear appearance. Spinal lipomas have similar MRI characteristics compared to subcutaneous fat without evidence of septations or nonfatty components [18]. They are usually dorsal to the spinal cord and well circumscribed [19]. T2 weighted images of spinal lipoma are also hyperintense and can help in cases associated with meningocele. An example of intradural lipoma visualized using T1 and T2 weighted MRI.

For patients in whom MRI is contraindicated, computed tomography myelography is the modality of choice [20]. It can show the anatomy of subarachnoid space but it is an invasive procedure and provides less information compared to MRI.

In cases of spinal lipomas in young infants with associated skin abnormalities, spinal ultrasonography could be used. Fat appears highly echogenic and intradural

Table 15.1 Characteristics of intradural lipomas using different imaging modalities [22]

Radiography	Hypodense mass, posterior elements are generally intact, canal widening due to bony erosions. Lumbosacral scoliosis could be seen in some patients.
Non-enhanced computed tomography	Hypodense intradural mass, focal and lobulated. There may be a widening of neural foramina at the level of the lipoma.
Myelography	Hypodense mass within the dura is partially surrounded by hyperdense contrast. Large lipomas could produce a spinal block.
Greyscale ultrasound	Echogenic mass, reduced conus medullaris motion. Used in infants for screening, if positive confirmation with MRI is needed.
T1 weighted MRI	Well-circumscribed hyperintense mass associated with the spinal cord. Decreased signal intensity on fat saturation sequences. Sagittal and axial t1w MRI is the standard to define lipoma extend and relations to surrounding tissues. In STIR, short tau inversion recovery, there is a decreased signal intensity confirming the fatty content
T2 weighted MRI	Similar appearance and signal intensity as T1W MRI.

fat can be easily detected. Spinal ultrasonography could be used to detect associated vertebral abnormalities and could be used to observe the motion of the spinal cord [21].

15.4.2 Gross Picture

The intradural lipoma specimen is soft in consistency, yellowish in color, glistening in appearance, and has a fusiform shape. It appears to be closely but non-invasively related to the posterior part of the spinal cord. Externally, the tumor is irregular, lobulated, and encapsulated. Usually, there is no exact cutting plane because of the involvement of many spinal cord segments [23] Fig. 15.1 shows an intradural extramedullary cervical cord lipoma after midline durotomy.

15.4.3 Microscopic Picture

Intradural lipoma is a heavily vascularized tumor of lobulated adipose tissue. It is made of a homogenous mass of mature fat cells divided by fibrous connective tissue among nervous tissue. Calcifications, myocytes, glial cells, or arachnoids may be found. The nerve bundles are situated near the specimen's margin, indicating subsequent entrapment of surrounding nerve roots by the lipoma. Fat cells are big, regular, and polygonal in shape with a soft pale cell membrane and eccentric nucleus [24] Fig. 15.1b shows the histopathological appearance of cervical intradural lipoma.

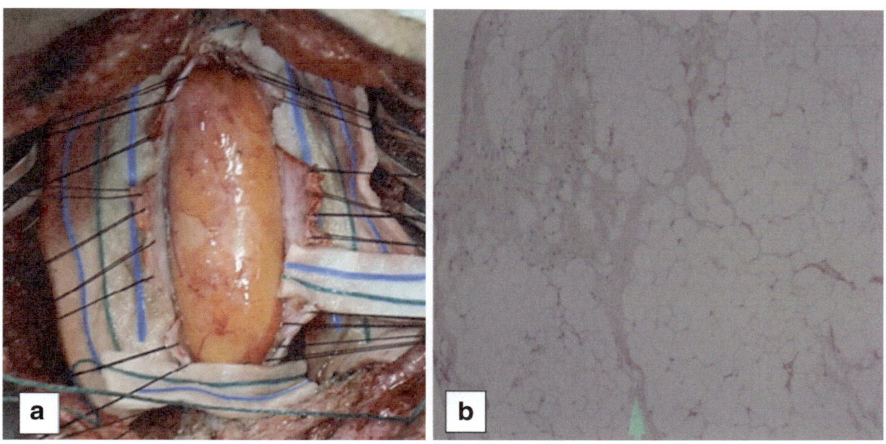

Fig. 15.1 (**a**) intradural lipomatous mass appearing after midline durotomy, (**b**) histopathological photograph showing the lipomatous cells with scattered dense connective tissue (arrow) [26].

These cells are a constituent of the fat storage in the body and may grow whenever fat is being deposited. Fat cells expand significantly throughout infancy so, minor lipomas in newborns may grow significantly during infancy and shrink if the patient loses weight. There are no malignancy or neoplastic characteristics like dedifferentiation, invasion, pleomorphism, or increased N/C ratio [25].

15.5 Clinical Presentation

15.5.1 Time of Presentation

55% of all patients seek medical attention in their second and third decades of life. Nearly 24% of patients present in their first decade, while 16% present in their fifth. Patients present in early infancy and childhood can show manifestations such as tetraplegia or floppy baby syndrome because of birth trauma to the spinal cord. Most people are symptomatic for at least 2 years before they seek medical care. Yet, more than 80% of cases with lipomas limited to the cervical spine may have symptoms for over 10 years [25].

15.5.2 Signs and Symptoms

Clinical pictures differ from one patient to another. Some may be asymptomatic, and others may develop worsening neurological symptoms secondary to the size of the lipoma.

Symptoms of intradural lipoma are produced by the mass's growth and its compression o the spinal cord while it grows because of fatter deposition in the lipoma. Patients often experience continuous and progressive deterioration as the tumor grows, which might result in nerve root displacement or crowding (tethering the cord) [1, 2].

The most common associated clinical manifestations are Numbness, spastic weakness in the limbs, bladder, and bowel incontinence. Back and leg pain is also possible. Radicular pain is unusual. Symptoms differ according to the location of the intradural lipoma (Fig. 15.2).

Most important signs and symptoms:

- Cervical and thoracic intradural lipoma: progressive ascending mono or paraparesis, stiffness, hypoesthesia, and deep sensory loss.
- Lumbosacral intradural lipoma: lower limb flaccid paralysis, bladder sphincter dysfunction
- Terminal intradural lipoma: Bowel/bladder malfunction, lower limb weakness, sensory impairment, foot deformity, scoliosis
- A sacral indentation or birthmark is often seen in patients with intradural lipomas [27, 28].

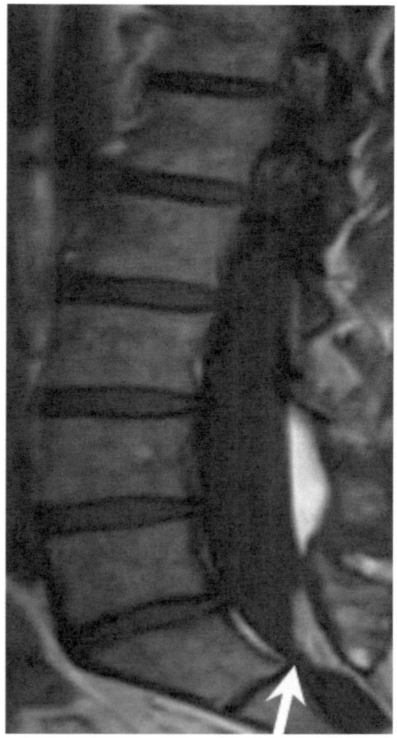

Fig. 15.2 A case of intradural spinal lipoma (arrow) with tethered spinal cord at the level of L5-S1, hyperintense on lumbar spine T1 weighted MRI [36]

15.5.3 Tethered Cord Syndrome

Spinal lipomatous malformation with an intradural component is commonly associated with tethered spinal cord syndrome [29]. Tethering is a condition where the spinal cord is fixed in a position lower than the second lumbar vertebra after development. When the child is born, the conus medullaris, the lower portion of the cord, is present at the level of L3 and ascends to L1 due to disproportionate growth between the spinal canal and the spinal cord. In the case of tethering, there is stretching of the nerves of the cauda equina and this stretch could lead to spinal cord damage which is exaggerated with spinal flexion. In addition to the mechanical effect of tethering, there may be reduced cord perfusion resulting in an ischemic injury to the conus [30]. Spinal lipomas could result in asymmetric tethering of the cord which leads to rotation and unequal development of the nerve roots [31]. Tethered cord syndrome is mostly associated with lipomas affecting the lumbosacral region and includes the symptoms of lower extremity weakness, leg pain, back pain, and urological symptoms such as sphincter dysfunction.

15.6 Management

15.6.1 Different Management Plans

There are many debates about the best management of intradural lipomas and there have been considerable variations in their therapy. This ranges from conservative care with rigorous dietary control to invasive entire lesion excision. The fat in the intradural lipoma is metabolically like normal body fat. Accordingly, many researchers advocate that controlling body weight may be a key component in the conservative management of patients with spinal intradural lipomas. These patients should then be put on intense weight loss and strict diet monitoring. Unfortunately, this is not necessarily the case since there have been recorded cases of fast lipoma growth in obese individuals despite strict dietary management. Anyway, the diet should be considered in obese patients [32].

15.6.2 The Goal of Surgery and the Best Surgical Technique

There are debates about the most appropriate surgical procedures in patients with intradural lipomas. The goal of any surgery is decompression of the spinal cord because clinical manifestations originate from spinal cord compression [33].

The primary surgical management plan consists of partial resection and duraplasty [34]. Duraplasty is very important to decrease the incidence of recurrence. Patients who undergo partial resection alone have more risk of recurrence. The surgery is usually performed with the aid of anesthesia and intraoperative electrophysiological monitoring (IONM). To separate the functional spinal cord from the bulk, intraoperative electrophysiological stimulation with evoked EMG monitoring is frequently employed. IONM is important in avoiding and anticipating permanent neurological deficits so that subsequent surgical measures can be adjusted. If patient symptoms continue to deteriorate after the surgery, more debulking and removal may be needed [34].

Here are the steps of the surgery:

1. The patient is set in a prone manner
2. c-arm serves to verify the level of lipoma and surgery, mostly using AP imaging.
3. The posterior midline is then opened, and dorsal vertebral components are removed (laminotomy is preferable).
4. After hemostasis is achieved, the dura is dissected using tagging stitches.
5. Following that, partial Lipoma debulking is performed with sharp dissection using either micro scissors and bipolar coagulation or CUSA (Cavitron Ultrasonic Surgical Aspirator). Co2 Laser can be used
6. Duraplasty is finally performed to close the dura
7. Neuromonitoring readings are taken many times between the steps

15.6.3 When to Do the Surgery

Surgery shouldn't be performed on asymptomatic patients. Cases that are asymptomatic or who only have local symptoms, such as pain, with no neurological manifestations should be conservatively handled with routine clinical and radiological monitoring.

Any case who experiences deteriorating local symptoms, such as increasing pain, or who develops any new neurological symptoms or signs, should be given surgical consideration. This is due to the possibility that in certain patients, the spinal cord may have reached a point where it can no longer accommodate the increasing mechanical pressure and there is no longer any physiological reserve. Neurological impairment quickly becomes apparent if decompression is not performed [25].

15.6.4 Prognosis and Sequela after Surgery

Improvements after surgery differ greatly from one patient to another. But frequently there is an improvement in pain, muscle weakness, hypoesthesia, and many other motor and sensory manifestations [32] However, most patients experience remaining neurological sequela following the surgery of intradural lipoma. Electromyography with nerve conduction study can be used for evaluating the extent of neural dysfunction which aids in evaluating the degree of post-operative recovery [35]. Rehabilitation and physiotherapy form important aspects of post-operative management. Congenital intradural lipoma might restrict the normal formation and development of the near spinal cord tissue. As a result, there may not be big improvements after surgery in many cases [33].

15.6.5 Total Resection Dangers and Extent of Lipoma Debulking

The aim of surgical resection is just debulking not total removal. Excision of total lipoma is very complicated because of the absence of cleavage plane, indolent nature of the lipoma, and mingling of neural and fat tissue [33].

Surgical hazards and the risks associated with complete excision have long been known. Patients who had a laminectomy and total resection reported disastrous postoperative paraplegia. The extent of lipoma removed and the percentage of the tumor debulked have nothing to do with the outcomes of the surgery. There was a patient who removed 70% of the lesion and neurologically worsened. Yet, another patient removed just 40% and had a neurological big improvement. There are reported cases with good outcomes with laminectomy and biopsy alone. Adjusting the amount of decompression necessary and the maintenance of neurological structures is important. The postsurgical neurological function can improve, even with a large residual neoplasm present [25].

15.7 Conclusion

A spinal cord lipoma is a fat within the normally positioned spinal cord. They are very rare lesions and form around 1% of all spinal tumors. They commonly occur with spinal dysraphism. Truly non-dysraphic spinal cord lipomas are quite uncommon. The exact etiology of spinal lipomas is still not thoroughly known, but the most accepted theory, the developmental error theory, states that the underlying mechanism is errors occurring during primary and secondary neurulation. Lumbosacral lipomas are commonly associated with spinal dysraphism. Non-dysraphic intradural lipomas are usually in the thoracic region followed by the cervical and cervico-dorsal regions. They usually involve several segments in the spinal cord. Clinical presentation of intradural lipoma range from asymptomatic to worsening neurological symptoms. They are produced by the mass's growth and its compression to the spinal cord. The most common associated clinical manifestations are pain, Numbness, spastic weakness in the limbs, bladder incontinence, and sensory loss. Multiple imaging modalities could be used to visualize intradural lipomas. Magnetic resonance imaging is the most sensitive imaging modality for diagnosing spinal lipomas and for planning surgeries. There is controversy about the best management of intradural lipoma. The aim of surgery is decompression of the spinal cord to ease the clinical manifestations. The primary surgery performed is partial resection of the lipoma with duroplasty. Total resection must be avoided. The extent of lipoma removed and the percentage of the tumor debulked have nothing to do with the outcomes of the surgery. Asymptomatic cases can be managed with routine clinical and radiological monitoring. There is evidence that diet and weight loss might help.

Multiple Choice Questions

1. **Which of the following is the most accepted theory for the underlying embryogenesis of spinal lipomas?**

   A. Developmental error theory.
   B. Metaplastic theory.
   C. Mesenchymal inhibition theory.
   D. Endocrinal theory.

2. **What is the broad term for the processes happening between primary and secondary neurulation.**

   A. Transitional neurulation
   B. Junctional neurulation

C. Intermediate neurulation
D. Middle neurulation

3. **According to pang classification for spinal lipomas, chaotic lipomas occur due to an error in:**

A. Primary neurulation
B. Early stage of secondary neurulation
C. Late stage of secondary neurulation
D. Transitional neurulation

4. **Which is the best imaging modality for visualizing spinal lipomas?**

A. MRI
B. CT
C. Ultrasonography.
D. X-ray

5. **On histopathological examination of a lipoma extracted from the spinal cord of the patient which of the following could be observed?**

A. Dedifferentiation
B. Increased N/C ratio
C. Pleomorphism
D. Regular fat cells with eccentric nucleus

6. **10 years old boy presented with difficulty in walking, weakness of both of his legs for the last 2 months. Clinical examination showed no hair, fistula, or mass on his spine. Neurological examination showed spastic paraplegia with diminished sensations. MRI showed a hyperintense mass between D3-D8 segments on the sagittal T1 and T2 weighted images. On Axial scan, the mass was found dorsal to the cord. Most likely the diagnosis is:**

A. Dermoid cyst.
B. Neuroepithelial cyst.
C. Intradural lipoma.
D. Meningocele.

7. **A mother of 8 years old girl came to the neurosurgery clinic. She said that her daughter was diagnosed with intradural lipoma, and it was large. She complained that the other doctor didn't want to remove the entire lesion. He told her that he was going to remove from 40–70% of it according to investigations the girl should do. The mother was angry at the doctor and thought he was an amateur and left his clinic immediately. She said that she is coming to you to remove the lipoma completely. What is the best thing that you can do?**

A. remove the entire lesion completely as the mother wishes
B. remove 50% of the lesion

C. explain to the mother that the aim of the surgery is just debulking not total resection so that her daughter clinical manifestations disappear
D. remove 70% of the lesion

8. **19-year-old male came to the clinic complaining from local back pain that hasn't increased but was always there for years. History taking revealed that a doctor prescribed him Orlistat (a weight loss drug) 2 months ago after his BMI became 30.0. There were no sensory or motor manifestation. After many investigations, he was diagnosed with intradural lipoma. What is the best management for him?**

   A. He can go home as there are no neurological manifestations
   B. He needs to go to surgery before the lipoma grow
   C. He just needs to continue taking his weight loss drug
   D. He needs rigorous dietary control with routine clinical and radiological monitoring.

9. **What is the best surgical technique for cases with symptomatic intradural spinal lipomas?**

   A. partial resection and duroplasty
   B. laminectomy and total resection
   C. laminectomy and biopsy
   D. intense diet

10. **In histopathological examination of extracted spinal intradural lipoma, structures of which embryological germ layers might be found?**

   A. Endoderm
   B. Ectoderm
   C. Mesoderm
   D. All the above

Answers and Explanation

1. The answer is (A): Developmental error theory is the most accepted theory to explain the etiology of spinal lipomas
2. The answer is (B): Primary and secondary neurulation are not separate entities but there is a continuity between the formed primary and secondary neural tubes. The processes happening between them were termed "junctional neurulation"
3. The answer is (B): A new class was added to PANG classification known as chaotic lipoma with its developmental origin occurring at junctional neurulation
4. The answer is (A): MRI is the best imaging modality for visualizing spinal lipomas
5. The answer is (D): Fat cells in the lipomas are part of the normal adipose tissue of body. They are big, regular, and polygonal in shape with a soft pale cell membrane and eccentric nucleus.
6. The answer is (C): clinical picture and imaging affirm that the diagnosis is intradural lipoma

7. The answer is (C): The extent of lipoma removed and the percentage of the tumor debulked have nothing to do with the outcomes of the surgery. Adjusting the amount of decompression necessary and the maintenance of neurological structures is important.
8. The answer is (D): many researchers advocate that controlling body weight may be a key component in the conservative management of patients with spinal intradural lipomas. Cases that are asymptomatic should be conservatively handled with routine clinical and radiological monitoring.
9. The answer is (A): partial resection and duroplasty is the best surgical technique for cases with symptomatic intradural spinal lipomas
10. The answer is (D): All three germ layers Ectoderm, mesoderm, and endoderm could be found in histopathological examination of extracted spinal intradural lipoma

References

1. Koen JL, McLendon RE, George TM. Intradural spinal teratoma: evidence for a dysembryogenic origin. Report of four cases. J Neurosurg [Internet]. 1998;89(5):844–51. [cited 2022 Aug 20]. Available from: https://pubmed.ncbi.nlm.nih.gov/9817426/
2. Naidich TP, Mclone DG, Mutluer S. A new understanding of dorsal dysraphism with lipoma (lipomyeloschisis): radiologic evaluation and surgical correction. 1983.; Available from: www.ajronline.org
3. Ammerman BJ, Henry JM, de Girolami U, Earle KM. Intradural lipomas of the a clinicopathological correlation spinal cord. J Neurosurg. 1976;44:331–6.
4. Nievelstein RAJ, Hartwig NG, Vermeij-Keers C, Valk J. Embryonic development of the mammalian caudal neural tube. Teratology [Internet]. 1993;48(1):21–31. [cited 2022 Aug 20]. Available from: https://pubmed.ncbi.nlm.nih.gov/8351645/
5. Dady A, Havis E, Escriou V, Catala M, Duband JL. Junctional neurulation: a unique developmental program shaping a discrete region of the spinal cord highly susceptible to neural tube defects. J Neurosci. 2014;34(39):13208–21.
6. Eibach S, Moes G, Hou YJ, Zovickian J, Pang D. Unjoined primary and secondary neural tubes: junctional neural tube defect, a new form of spinal dysraphism caused by disturbance of junctional neurulation. Childs Nerv Syst. 2017;33(10):1633–47. [cited 2022 Aug 20]. Available from: https://pubmed.ncbi.nlm.nih.gov/27796548/
7. Matsui H, Kanamori M, Miaki K. Expansive laminoplasty for lumbar intradural lipoma
8. Heon Kim C, Wang KC, Kim SK, Chung YN, Choi YL, Chi JG, et al. Spinal intramedullary lipoma: report of three cases. Spinal Cord. 2003;41(5):310–5.
9. Chapman PH. Congenital intraspinal lipomas: anatomic considerations and surgical treatment. Childs Brain. 1982;9(1):37–47.
10. Neurochirurgica A, Arai H, Sato K, Okuda O, Miyajima M, Hishii M, et al. Surgical experience of 120 patients with lumbosacral lipomas. 2001.
11. Pang D, Zovickian J, Oviedo A. Long-term outcome of total and near-total resection of spinal cord lipomas and radical reconstruction of the neural placode: part I - surgical technique. Neurosurgery. 2009;65(3):511–28.
12. Pang D, Zovickian J, Wong ST, Hou YJ, Moes GS, et al. Surgical treatment of complex spinal cord lipomas.
13. Morota N, Ihara S, Ogiwara H. New classification of spinal lipomas based on embryonic stage. J Neurosurg Pediatr. 2017;19(4):428–39.

14. Lee M, Rezai AR, Abbott R, Coelho DH, Epstein FJ. Intramedullary spinal cord lipomas. J Neurosurg. 1995;82(3):394–400. [cited 2022 Aug 23]. Available from: https://pubmed.ncbi.nlm.nih.gov/7861216/
15. Massimi L, Feitosa Chaves TM, Legninda Sop FY, Frassanito P, Tamburrini G, Caldarelli M. Acute presentations of intradural lipomas: case reports and a review of the literature. BMC Neurol. 2019;19(1) [cited 2022 Aug 23]. Available from: /pmc/articles/PMC6688213/.
16. Drapkin AJ. High cervical intradural lipoma. J Neurosurg [Internet]. 1974;41(6):699–704. [cited 2022 Aug 23]. Available from: https://pubmed.ncbi.nlm.nih.gov/4417026/
17. Kabir SMR, Thompson D, Rezajooi K, Casey ATH. Non-dysraphic intradural spinal cord lipoma: case series, literature review and guidelines for management. Acta Neurochir. 2010;152(7):1139–44.
18. Beall DP, Googe DJ, Emery RL, Thompson DB, Campbell SE, Ly JQ, et al. Extramedullary intradural spinal tumors: a pictorial review. Curr Probl Diagn Radiol. 2007;36:185–98.
19. Vasudha Patwardhan, Tufail Patanakar. MR imaging findings of intramedullary lipomas [Internet]. Available from: www.ajronline.org
20. Finn MA, Walker ML. Spinal lipomas: clinical spectrum, embryology, and treatment. Neurosurg Focus. 2007;23:1–12.
21. Caffey J, Naidich TP, Fernbach SK, Mclone DG, Shkolnik A. Sonography of the caudal award spine and back: congenital anomalies in children [Internet]. 1984. Available from: www.ajronline.org
22. Ross J, Moore K. Diagnostic imaging: spine. 3rd ed. Elsevier; 2015.
23. A. C, Dickman, Michael G. Fehlings ZLG. Spinal cord and spinal cord tumors. Am J Neuroradiol 2007.
24. Hanft S, Mccormick PC. Tumors of the spinal canal. In: Mehta AI, editor. Tumors of the spinal canal. New York: Thieme Medical Publishers, Inc.; 2022.
25. M.A.Hayat. Tumors of the central nervous system.
26. Panagopoulos D, Markogiannakis G, Koutzoglou M. Intradural–extramedullary cervical cord lipoma: case report and literature review. World Neurosurg. 2018;110:162–8.
27. Moore KR, Ross JS. Diagnostic imaging: spine, vol. 27. p. 1680–6.
28. Milla SS, Bixby SD. The teaching files. Pediatric.
29. Rhodes RH. Congenital spinal lipomatous malformations. Part 1. Spinal lipomas, lipomyeloceles, and lipomyelomeningoceles. Fetal Pediatr Pathol. 2020;39:194–245.
30. Warder DE. Tethered cord syndrome and occult spinal dysraphism. Neurosurg Focus. 2001;10(1) [cited 2022 Aug 24]. Available from: https://pubmed.ncbi.nlm.nih.gov/16749753/
31. Pierre-Kahn A, Lacombe J, Pichon J, Giudicelli Y, Renier D, Sainte-Rose C, et al. Intraspinal lipomas with spina bifida. Prognosis and treatment in 73 cases. J Neurosurg [Internet]. 1986;65(6):756–61. [cited 2022 Aug 24]. Available from: https://pubmed.ncbi.nlm.nih.gov/3534161/
32. Azzazi A, Sedik M, Sakr S. Surgical management for intradural spinal lipoma in adult patients without spinal dysraphism. Neurosurg Q. 2010;20(3):130–5.
33. Chung CK. Surgery of spinal cord tumors based on anatomy. 2021.
34. Ikeda N, Odate S, Shikata J, Yamamura S, Kawaguchi S. Surgical strategies and outcomes for intradural lipomas over the past 20 years. J Clin Neurosci. 2019;1(60):107–11.
35. Alexiou G, Prodromou N. Pediatric neurosurgery for clinicians; 2022. p. 185–201.
36. Horrion J, Houbart MA, Georgiopoulos A, Bottosso N. Adult intradural lipoma with tethered spinal cord syndrome. JBR-BTR [Internet]. 2014;97(2):121. [cited 2022 Aug 24]. Available from: https://pubmed.ncbi.nlm.nih.gov/25073248/

Chapter 16
Filum Lipoma

Yasser F. Almealawy, Jaafar I. Twayej, and Mohammed H. Al-Rammahi

Test your learning and check your understanding of this book's contents: use the "Springer Nature Flashcards" app to access questions using ▶ https://sn.pub/QCsfpd.
To use the app, please follow the instructions in Chap. 1

16.1 Introduction

Spinal lipoma is one of the congenital abnormalities that affects the spinal cord [1], it is a grouping of spinal malformation that have been loosely grouped together by the percutaneous lesion they countenance [2].

("the suffix "oma" is used to described a neoplastic event involving in pathophysiology of a lesion [2]"). Lipomas of spine are two types: the conus medullaris and the filum terminate, both called as lumbosacral lipomas. Disorders of embryogenesis can give rise to some of these lipomas. This chapter is going to discuss the filum lipoma.

Y. F. Almealawy (✉)
Department of Medicine, Medical Student, University of Kufa, Najaf, Iraq

J. I. Twayej
Department of Medicine, 2022 Graduate of College of Medicine, University of Kufa, Najaf, Iraq

M. H. Al-Rammahi
Department of Neurosurgery, 2021 Graduate of College of Medicine, University of Kufa, Najaf, Iraq

K. F. AlAli, H. T. Hashim (eds.), *Congenital Spine Malformations*, https://doi.org/10.1007/978-3-031-59031-3_16

("Filum terminale has been termed "The unpaired nerve", because it is what remains of the spinal cord at the end of the coccyx, was described by Galen [3]"). ("Newer studies rather explain filum terminale as a fibrovascular band attachment of the spinal cord to the coccyx [3]"). The filum lipoma is simply a fibrolipomatous thickening of the filum terminale [2].

Most patients with filar lipoma are asymptomatic (95%). Thus, clear estimation of the prevalence of the disease remains unknown [3].

16.1.1 Embryology and Pathogenesis

Normal spinal cord development occurs in three stages. The gastrulation is the first which takes place during (2–3 week). In this stage, the embryonic disc transfers from being a bilaminar disc to a trilaminar disc, which composed of ectoderm, endoderm and mesoderm.

The primary neurulation is second stage which happens around third or fourth week. The neural plate formation by the interaction between notochord and ectoderm, then, the primary tube formation by bends and folds of the neural plate.

The third stage and the last is the secondary neurulation phase taking place around fifth and sixth weeks. In this stage, the caudal cells migrate to form secondary neural tube [4]. Which then undergo cavitation to form filum terminate.

Defect or abnormality happening in one of any steps can cause spinal cord malformation.

Spinal dysraphism is categorized into an open type, which has a defect in the skin that covers the tissue of neural leading to its exposure to the environment, and a closed type where the overlying skin is intact [4].

Filum lipoma and tight filum terminale are simple close dysraphism without any subcutaneous mass.

Filar lipomas, however, are considered fibrolipomatous. They originate from various tissues including ectodermal, mesodermal and endodermal tissues. Most frequent were from mesodermal origin, same as vessels, kidneys, cartilage, and neurosensorial corpuscle [5].

Normally the disjunction or detachment of the cutaneous ectoderm from the neural ectoderm is complete [6], and there is also closure of neural tube [4]. Filum lipoma occurs because of an abnormality of secondary neurulation. There will be an impairment of canalization and the mature cells that are capable of maturing into adipocyte to be involved in formation of filum lipoma [2, 7]. "In filum terminale there is "premature disjunction" that occurs in neural tube from the surrounding ectoderm. This non-disjunction makes the neural tube open posteriorly and allowing mesenchymal cells to enter the cleft. These cells are stimulated by primitive ependyma to form fatty tissue" [6].

16.2 Anatomy of Filum Terminate

In adults, the filum terminates located at the middle third body of first lumbar (L1). The level of spinal cord termination is sometimes lower to L3.

It consists from Internum and Extremum, The Internum, the upper intradural component, is covered by spinal dura and arachnoid meninges and consists of glial and ependymal cells and is 15 cm in length.

The extremum, which is the lower intradural component, fuses with dura mater and attaches inferiorly to dorsal coccyx and is 5 cm in length.

The filum terminale extremum was measured to about 2.2 cm in newborn and 7.5 cm in adults. It is made up of a fibrous tissue that continues with that of pia mater and is surrounded by dura mater.

16.3 Biochemistry

The normal function of the adipose tissue is to store lipid and metabolize lipids in response to hormonal and metabolic stimulations. An increase in lipid storage and a reduction in lipid mobilization and can lead to the promotion of fat.

The lipoprotein lipase (LPL) and insulin control lipogenesis and lipid storage. On the other side, lipolysis is promoted by catecholamines (adenylate cyclase and cyclic AMP) [5]. These catecholamines bind to two different adrenergic receptors which are alpha 2 receptor and beta receptor. Alpha receptors stimulation causes inhibition of adenylate cyclase, cyclic AMP and lipolysis. Beta receptor stimulation the opposite to that [1].

In summary, lipogenesis is mediated by LPL and insulin while lipolysis is mediated by adenylate cyclase and cyclic AMP.

We need to distinguish between fat cells from normal adipose tissue and from congenital intraspinal lipoma. Studies show that the metabolic activities were similar in both of intraspinal lipoma and normal adipose tissue [5].

16.4 Histology and Histopathology

Lipomas are made of mature clustered adipocytes separated by collagen bands. These adipocytes are arranged in lobules with loose connective tissue.

Intraspinal lipomas are composed of normal adipocytes, however, we also know that normal adipocytes are capable of increasing and decreasing their growth along the rest of the fatty pool [5]. The same occurs in intraspinal lipomas because as we explored that it is composed of mature and normal adipocytes.

Epidural fat capable of growth and cause spinal cord compression, and this epidural fat is comparable to normal adipose tissue [5].

Studies show lipomas are different from lipomatous. Latter are benign and slowly growing fat with increase in lipogenic activity and defective lipolytic activity [5], while the filum lipoma are benign, overgrowth of fat cells.

In normal adults, the incidental fat within filum terminale is about 17%.

It is theorized that the tension of infiltrates may lead to subsequent neuronal dysfunction and impaired mitochondrial oxidative metabolism that result in stretching of the cauda equina [3].

16.5 Clinical Features

Lipomas of the filum terminale can be incidental findings in many individuals [8]. That is why many patients may actually have the condition but are in fact asymptomatic. A fatty filum terminale that is not enlarged in an asymptomatic patient can be even considered a normal variant [9].

When patients present clinically with symptoms, these will be attributed to tethered cord syndrome (TCS). In fact, lumbosacral lipomas are a very common congenital cause of tethered cord syndrome [10]. It is when the conus medularis is tethered and stretched by the thickened filum terminale causing various neurological manifestations. This most commonly occur during periods of rapid growth especially during adolescence, 5 to 15 years of age [11]. In fact, thickened filum is the most common cause for tethered cord syndrome [12]. Symptoms can also arise for the first time in adults following abrupt flexion movements, such as abdominal flexion, motor vehicle accidents and prolonged positioning in lithotomy position during delivery [13].

The most commonly recorded symptoms include pain (80% of patients), sensory disturbance (78%), weakness (70%), and urinary disturbance (68%). Almost all patients complained of neurological symptoms (98.5). Pain was predominantly located around the perineal and gluteal areas, in addition to leg pain that did not follow specific dermatomal distribution. Regarding sensory disturbance, it also mostly affected the saddle region and distal lower limbs with patchy distribution. Lower extremities are also the ones usually affected with weakness, although it would be disproportionate and accompanied by hyperreflexia and spasticity. Spasticity can manifest when the foot is turned inside as the child is sitting. Sometimes, subtle signs of deficit can manifest as difficulty in performing tasks such as riding a bicycle, or falling during running and playing sports. Urinary symptoms tend to occur equally in pediatrics and adults4; however, specific manifestations may differ. For example, children complain of weak urinary stream and enuresis, while adults report urgency and stress incontinence [14]. Other urinary features include detrusor hyperreflexia poor bladder compliance, dyssnergia and decreased sensation. All of these can contribute to chronic urinary tract infections in these patients. The problem with urological manifestations is that their diagnosis in infants and children is difficult as they might be socially embarrassing. Fecal incontinence can coexist with urological symptoms, and even exacerbating them10. Patients may sometimes exhibit cutaneous manifestations at the lumbar and sacral regions. These can include lipoma, hypertrichosis, hemangioma and dimples). Orthopaedic findings are also present and they include cavovarus foot, length discrepancies of the lower limbs [15].

16.6 Investigations

In imaging, the normal filum terminale can barely be seen. The test of choice would of course be magnetic resonance imaging (MRI). It has been suggested that the threshold of diagnosis of thickened filum is 2 mm [3, 16]. Also, the thick filum would appear hyperintense among the CSF in T1 images [17]. However, a common difficulty in diagnosis arises in the fact that many cases where there is fat in the filum are only incidental and normal (up to 6%)9, and tethering of the cord may never actually occur in them. Therefore, it is important to bear in mind when diagnosing filar lipoma both the clinical and radiological findings. Austinite and associates studied cases of TCS between 1936 and 2007, and they found that 7.9% of those had their level of conus at or above L2-L3 [12]. The conus is considered to be low if it is bellow L2 vertebral level, and the conus medullaris is found to be more posterior than normal. In that case, the filum may be in contact with the dura at L5 vertebral level. With these criteria in mind, tethered cord syndrome can be diagnosed [17].

Another thing to investigate while studying the spine is the spinal cord. It is imperative to exclude the presence of associated anomalies such as split cord syndrome. In infants, ultrasonography can be used to identify the level of the cord, diagnose intraspinal lipomas and exclude associated spinal dysraphism. Its use, however, is limited to infant's bellow 6 months of age so as to well visualize the spinal cord [10].

Patients need to undergo urodynamic testing as it has been found that bladder dysfunction can precede other clinical signs [18]. As the interpretation of urodynamic results is difficult in young children, the most useful parameters are the altered bladder volume, bladder-sphincter synergy and the activity of detrusor muscles.

CT scanning is of limited use, and is of benefit when MRI is contraindicated. If myelography and CT were obtained, thick filum would appear as small round filling defects extending through multiple sections [17].

16.7 Classification and Grading

The classification of FL is based on whether the conus medullaris is at a normal age-specific position or not in addition to the presence of symptoms (neurological manifestations). Therefore, there are four grades. However, the following classification is not considering the thickness of the filum or the presence of spina bifid [11].

16.8 Management

Surgical intervention is the choice. Generally, symptomatic patients with low-lying conus medullaris should undergo detethering procedure. However, in asymptomatic patients with low-lying conus medullaris, prophylactic surgical detethering should only be done if family requests and risks should be clearly addressed. In symptomatic cases with normal thickness filum terminale and normal position, conus medullaris surgical detethering is indicated.

16.9 Surgical Approach (Interlaminar Approach)

It is the sectioning of the thickened filum terminale which interrupts the connection between the conus medullaris and fat-infiltrated and hypertrophied filum. One of the essential steps in the surgery is to identify the filum from the surrounding roots. It looks greyer and larger. However, intraoperative monitoring will provide better certainty by monitoring the electromyographic activity of the lower limb and external anal sphincter activity. After induction of the anesthesia, the patient rolled to a prone position. The next step is to Prepare and sterilize the surgical field (lumbar region) with I.V antibiotics followed by a midline lumbar incision of about 1.5 cm. The surgeon stands on the left side of the patient. It is followed by removing the paraspinous muscle by inserting a periosteal elevator. Then, an extension of the dissection to the inter-spinous ligament to expose the ligamentum flavum. L5-S1 or L4-L5 interlaminar spaces are exposed using a skin hook. A mid-point incision of the ligamentum flavum followed by medial retraction of the falvum using sutures to expose the epidural fat. After removing the fat and incising the dura followed by the arachnoid membrane the fatty filum is identified. Stimulating the identified structure with no electromyographic activity confirms it is the fatty filum. After the fatty filum is coagulated and sectioned, the dural sac and arachnoid membrane are closed. Followed by restoring the epidural fat and wound closure.

The postoperative wound-related complications and new neurological deficits are uncommon complication.

16.10 Prognosis

It is suggested that neurological deficit would likely occur in young patients rather than older ones. In a study done by Bulsara et al., the distance of the filum to the conus medullaris was found to be more associated with clinical features than the thickness of the filum. 13 mm distance was most predicative of neurological presentation, with significant statistics [19].

Overall, filar lipoma is considered a benign disease. Its treatment, especially the prophylactic method, carries significantly better prognosis with low complication rate [9].

Multiple Choice Questions

1. **The neural tube opens posteriorly and allowing mesenchymal cells to enter the cleft due to:**

   A. abnormality of secondary neurulation
   B. premature disjunction
   C. complete disjunction
   D. abnormality of gastrulation

2. **The upper intradural components (the Internum) are:**

   A. attached inferiorly to dorsal coccyx
   B. covered by spinal dura and fuses with dura mater
   C. consist from ependymal cell only
   D. covered by spinal dura and arachnoid meninges and 15 cm in length

3. **A 10-year-old girl presented to the GP with pain on the right lower limb. Her mother reports no recent events of trauma. The child's past medical history is negative for any serious illness, apart from the common flu. On examination, she is calm and cooperative. It is noticed that she has some sensory loss in her right lower leg, with some weakness in the left. MRI scans of the lumbar spine show hyperintensity of the filum terminale. She is referred to the neurosurgeon, who advises the family with surgery to detether the cord. Prior to performing the operation, which further diagnostic test is needed for this patient?**

   A. CT scan of the spine
   B. Lumbar puncture for cytology and culture
   C. Urodynamic studies
   D. Electromyography of the right upper limb
   E. Electroencephalography

4. **Which of the following is the most common cause for tethered cord syndrome?**

   A. Lumbosacral lipomas
   B. Lipomyelomeningocele
   C. Tethering adhesions after spinal surgery
   D. Diastematomyelia

5. **Filar lipomas are most often diagnosed at presentation.**

   A. True?
   B. False?

Answers

1) ***B***

   Because the Filum lipoma occurs due to premature disjunction that makes neural tube open posteriorly and allow the primitive ependyma to form fatty tissue.
2) ***D***

   The Internum or upper intradural component are covered by spinal dura and arachnoid meninges while the lower is fuses with dura mater and attached inferiorly to dorsal coccyx.
3) ***C***

   It has been found that many patients with tethered cord syndrome have abnormal urodynamics even prior to other clinical symptoms. It is therefore essential in this patient to assess her lower urinary tract functions in order to establish baseline indices for further follow up and possible treatment.
4) ***A***

   Lumbosacral lipomas.
5) ***B***

   Filar lipomas are common and are mostly incidental findings.

References

1. Di Rocco C, Pang D, Rutka J. Textbook of pediatric neurosurgery. Cham: Springer International Publishing; 2020.
2. Trapp B, de Andrade Lourenção Freddi T, de Oliveira Morais Hans M, Fonseca Teixeira Lemos Calixto I, Fujino E, Alves Rojas LC, Dalul Gomez G. A practical approach to diagnosis of spinal dysraphism. Radiographics. 2021;41(2):559–75.
3. Tubbs RS, Oskouian RJ, Blount JP, Oakes WJ. Occult spinal dysraphism. Cham, Switzerland: Springer Nature; 2019.
4. Rufener SL, Ibrahim M, Raybaud CA, Parmar HA. Congenital spine and spinal cord malformations—pictorial review. Am J Roentgenol. 2010;194(3_supplement):S26–37.
5. Pierre-Kahn A, Zerah M, Renier D, Cinalli G, Sainte-Rose C, Lellouch-Tubiana A, Brunelle F, Le Merrer M, Giudicelli Y, Pichon J, Kleinknecht B, Nataf F. Congenital lumbosacral lipomas. Childs Nerv Syst. 1997;13(6):298–334.; discussion 335. https://doi.org/10.1007/s003810050090.
6. Morioka T, Murakami N, Shimogawa T, Mukae N, Hashiguchi K, Suzuki SO, Iihara K. Neurosurgical management and pathology of lumbosacral lipomas with tethered cord. Neuropathology. 2017;37:385–92.
7. Rossi A, Biancheri R, Cama A, Piatelli G, Ravegnani M, Tortori-Donati P. Imaging in spine and spinal cord malformations. Eur J Radiol. 2004;50(2):177–200.
8. Brown E, Matthes JC, Bazan C 3rd, Jinkins JR. Prevalence of incidental intraspinal lipoma of the lumbosacral spine as determined by MRI. Spine (Phila Pa 1976). 1994;19(7):833–6. https://doi.org/10.1097/00007632-199404000-00018.
9. Poe, L. B. (2020). Tight filum syndrome. Radsource. Accessed 27 Aug 2022, from https://radsource.us/tight-filum-syndrome/#:~:text=Fibrolipomas%20of%20the%20filum%20terminale,and%20the%20tight%20filum%20syndrome.
10. Kim DH, Betz RR, Huhn SL, Newton P. Surgery of the pediatric spine. New York, NY: Thieme; 2008.

11. Blount JP, Elton S. Spinal lipomas. Neurosurg Focus. 2001;10(1):1–13. https://doi.org/10.3171/foc.2001.10.1.4.
12. Aufschnaiter K, Fellner F, Wurm G. Surgery in adult onset tethered cord syndrome (ATCS): review of literature on occasion of an exceptional case. Neurosurg Rev. 2008;31:371–83. discussion 384
13. Pinto FC, Fontes RB, Mde L, Amodio DT, Porro FF, Machado J. Anatomic study of the filum terminale and its correlations with the tethered cord syndrome. Neurosurgery. 2002;51(3):725–30.
14. Giddens JL, Radomski SB, Hirshberg ED, et al. Urodynamic findings in adults with the tethered cord syndrome. J Urol. 1999;161:1249–54.
15. Yundt KD, Park TS, Kaufman BA. Normal diameter of filum terminate in children: in vivo measurement. Pediatr Neurosurg. 1997;27(5):257–9.
16. Hoffman HJ, Hendrick EB, Humphreys RP. The tethered spinal cord: its protean manifestations, diagnosis and surgical correction. Childs Brain. 1976;2(3):145–55. https://doi.org/10.1159/000119610. PMID: 786565
17. La Marca F, Grant JA, Tomita T, McLone DG. Spinal lipomas in children: outcome of 270 procedures. Pediatr Neurosurg. 1997;26(1):8–16.
18. Vernet O, Farmer JP, Houle AM, et al. Impact of urodynamic studies on the surgical management of spinal cord tethering. J Neurosurg. 1996;85:555–9.
19. Bulsara KR, Zomorodi AR, Enterline DS, George TM. The value of magnetic resonance imaging in the evaluation of fatty filum terminale. Neurosurgery. 2004;54(2):375–9.

Chapter 17
Tight Filum Terminale

Ahmad Rjoub, Motaz Daraghma, and Yazan Demaidi

> Test your learning and check your understanding of this book's contents: use the "Springer Nature Flashcards" app to access questions using ▶ https://sn.pub/QCsfpd.
> To use the app, please follow the instructions in Chap. 1

17.1 Introduction

The Filum Terminale is a thin band of fibrous tissue that attaches the spinal cord to the coccyx [1, 2]. Previously, the filum terminale and its structure were not well studied or investigated until the beginning of the twentieth century, when it started to become an area of study due to the importance of its structure that is related to some neurological diseases [3]. Understanding the Tethered cord syndrome, which is detailed below, requires a thorough knowledge of embryology and the structure of the filum terminale. The filum terminale consists mainly of ependymal and glial cells and it measures about 20 cm in length, and it reaches the dorsal surface of the coccyx from the conus medullaris' tip [4]. According to some studies, the filum terminale contains neuronal stem cells and peripheral nerve cells, which may be used in transplantation in the future [5, 6]. It is divided into two parts: a distal extradural part called as the filum terminale externum and a proximal intradural part

---

The original version of the chapter has been revised. A correction to this chapter can be found at https://doi.org/10.1007/978-3-031-59031-3_23

A. Rjoub (✉) · Y. Demaidi
Department of Medicine, An-Najah National University, Nablus, Palestine

M. Daraghma
Faculty of Medicine, Arab American University of Palestine, Jenin, Palestine

K. F. AlAli, H. T. Hashim (eds.), *Congenital Spine Malformations*,
https://doi.org/10.1007/978-3-031-59031-3_17

called as the filum terminale internum. The proximal part of the filum terminale passes along with extensions from the arachnoid and dura mater and it measures about 15 cm [7]. The subarachnoid space that encompasses the filum terminale internum serves as the source of the Cerebrospinal Fluid (CSF) that is accessed by the lumber puncture [7]. The lower or distal part of the filum terminale is also described as the coccygeal ligament and is devoted to the dura mater. It is approximately 5 cm long [3]. The filum terminale is encircled by a gleaming connective tissue sheath that is connected proximally with the pia mater [3]. The filum terminale thickness varies along its course and is decreasing caudally. At its origin from the conus medullaris, the normal diameter of the filum terminale ranges from 0.4 to 2.5 mm, with a mean of 1.38 mm; while at its midpoint, the filum terminale diameter ranges from 0.10 to 1.55 mm, with an average diameter of 0.76 mm; and at the level of L5 to S1, the diameter of the filum terminale should be 1 mm or less [2]. Tight filum terminale is a term used to describe a filum terminale that has an abnormal structure resulting in tension and traction of the lower segments of the spinal cord leading to the signs and symptoms of the Tethered Cord Syndrome (TCS), which is then called Tight filum terminale syndrome [8, 9].

Tethered Cord Syndrome (TCS) could be primary or secondary TCS, which may be totally different forms [10]. While the abnormal tissue attachments of the spinal cord remain as the major pathogenic factor in the development of the primary TCS [10], TCS is the clinical entity that comprises a functional disorder due to tension in and traction to the lower spinal cord that causes a neuronal dysfunction in the lumbosacral region [11]. Tethered cord syndrome has traditionally been linked with a low conus medullaris under the level of L2 vertebra, as well as a thickened filum terminale in some patients [3, 12]. On the other hand, there were some reported cases of typical clinical presentation of TCS with imaging showing conus medullaris that is normally located and/or a normal diameter of the filum terminale "non-thickened", which is then called occult tight film terminale syndrome [9, 10, 13–16]. Secondary forms of TCS may be caused by or associated with myelomeningocele, lipoma, post-surgical repair of myelomeningocele or spina bifida, infection, or trauma to the spinal cord [2]. About 20–50% of children with repaired spina bifida defects require subsequent surgery later on in life to relief a tethered spinal cord according to the American Association of Neurological Surgeons [17]. TCS remains challenging to physicians in terms of diagnosis and treatment, but neurosurgeons play the main role in the management of TCS [2]. The pathogenesis of Tight filum terminale syndrome, its clinical features, its diagnosis, and its management are discussed in the following sections.

17.2 Pathophysiology

Under normal circumstances, the filum terminale anchors the spinal cord from the conus medullaris to the coccyx, and the elasticity of the filum terminale permits the lumbosacral cord to move slightly during the spine extension and flexion movements. Losing the filum terminale's elastic properties may put aberrant traction or strain the lumbosacral cord, especially with spine movement, leading to neuronal dysfunction [13, 18, 19]. Understanding the pathophysiological mechanisms of the tight filum terminal syndrome plays an important role in addressing the clinical symptoms of this syndrome, and providing indications for diagnostic studies or surgical procedures.

The tight filum terminale likely results from deviant involution in the form of apoptosis and/or necrosis of the terminal cord and fibers that form the filum terminale [2]. According to the literature, this is accompanied by fibrous and/or fatty tissue infiltration of the filum terminale, resulting in inelastic tight filum terminale that causes cord tethering [18, 20]. In the filum terminale of the patient with tethered cord syndrome, abnormally dense fibrous connective tissue has been observed in several histopathological studies [21, 22]. Shortening of the film terminale causes tethering of the spinal cord as discussed earlier. Yet, due to the presence of the dentate ligaments clamping the cord anteriorly to the T12 vertebra, the tethering effect is limited to the lumbosacral cord and especially the conus medullaris, so the clinical symptoms of tight filum terminale syndrome are limited to lower extremities sensory and motor deficits, urinary bladder incontinence, and bowels symptoms [18, 23, 24]. The clinical symptoms of this syndrome are believed to be caused by the stretching of nerve fibers, resulting in anomalous oxidative metabolism in the lumbosacral cord and nerve roots [23, 25].

The following concepts underlie the spinal cord stretching-induced alterations in the oxidative metabolism of spinal cord tissue. The Central Nervous System (CNS) tissue cells have higher energy requirements in the form of Adenosine triphosphate (ATP) and are totally dependent on the oxidative metabolism to generate an adequate amount of ATP to maintain the transmembrane ion gradient, electrical activity and signals transmission, the survival of the cells, and performing all the functions of the cells in the CNS. This is observed in multiple neurological dysfunctions, as minor periods of hypoxia or minimal changes in the oxidative metabolism cause significant neuronal cell death resulting in severe neurological impairments [18, 23, 24]. Several studies on human subjects as well as experimental studies on animal hypoxemia and spinal cord ischemia models displayed a strong correlation between the impairment of the oxidative metabolism and electrical activity in the lumbosacral segment of the spinal cord and the pathophysiology of the Tethered cord syndrome caused by tight filum terminale [18, 23, 24]. The studies on animal models showed that in periods of induced hypoxia, the interneuronal electrical activity decreases and sometimes disappears [18, 23, 24]. These experimental studies and the studies on human subjects before and after the untethering surgery showed a parallel correlation between the degree of oxidative metabolism impairment in cord tethering and clinical findings (neurological impairments), as patients with mild to moderate traction (mild to moderate neurological deficit) before the surgery showed mild to complete improvement after the surgery. While patients with severe neurological deficits before the surgery had only minimal improvement after the surgery [18, 23, 24].

It was observed that incontinence becomes irreparable before motor or sensory impairment. This is because the fact that the most sensitive part of the lumbosacral cord to traction is the conus medullaris, due to its proximity to the distal fixation of the cord, as well as its small diameter which is the smallest diameter found in the spinal cord. Stretching the conus medullaris stretching repeatedly causes early histologic damage that results in irreversible incontinence [24, 25]. As a result of intramedullary tension brought on by cord traction or tethering, the paravertebral muscles adjust reflexively (functionally) to change the curvature of the spinal column, allowing the spinal cord to travel through the spinal column for a shorter distance and reducing intramedullary tension. Scoliosis, high-arched feet, excessive lumbosacral lordosis, and hammer toes are some of the musculoskeletal malformations that result from this reflexive adjustment [24].

17.3 Diagnosis

17.3.1 Clinical Presentation

There is a wide range of symptoms of tight filum terminale syndrome (TFTS). A typical clinical sign of TFTS is spinal stiffness. Additionally, symptoms result from abnormalities in different body systems. The most common systems that are affected are the neurological, musculoskeletal, dermatological, and urinary systems. Bladder-bowel dysfunction, frequent urination, urgency, retention, incontinence, and recurrent urinary infections are all examples of urinary abnormalities. Neurological abnormalities can involve sensory dysfunction as well as motor dysfunction in upper and lower motor neurons, with motor deficits being more common than sensory deficits. The most common motor neurological manifestations include decreased strength, spasticity, atrophic changes, and poor gait development. When sensory dysfunction is present, back and/or leg pain are the most common symptoms that patients suffer from. Also, sensory dysfunction may affect the perineal area and the foot, which is why many undetected foot injuries, such as ulcers, occur. Scoliosis, deformity or asymmetry of the foot, limb-length disparity, calf asymmetry, and gluteal fold asymmetry are the most common orthopedic abnormalities that are associated with TFTS. Abnormal gluteal clefts, lumbosacral dimples, and hemangiomas are among the dermatological manifestations of TFTS. Interestingly, many asymptomatic tight filum terminale syndrome cases were incidentally discovered during neuroimaging. Depending on the clinical history and physical examination, bladder dysfunction in pediatric patients might be difficult to determine, and assessing the progress postoperatively can be difficult without an objective scale [13, 26, 27]. The clinical features of the TFTS are summarized in Table 17.1.

17.3.2 Neuroimaging

Different diagnosis modalities are used in the evaluation of TFTS, including Magnetic Resonance Imaging (MRI), X-rays, Computed Tomography Scan (CT scan), and urodynamic tests. Hence, plain or conventional X-rays are used in scoliotic deformity evaluation as part of the preoperative planning and assessment and

Table 17.1 Clinical features of tight filum terminale syndrome

Neurologic manifestations:
o Back pain or leg pain. o Abnormal gait. o Decreased strength. o Decreased sensation.
Orthopedic manifestations:
o Limb-length disparity. o Asymmetric feet. o Calves' asymmetry. o Scoliosis.
Dermatologic manifestations:
o Sacral dimple. o Abnormal gluteal cleft. o Hemangioma.
Urologic manifestations:
o Urinary incontinence. o Frequency. o Urgency. o Urinary retention.

are not used specifically for the diagnosis of TFTS. The general methods used in the diagnosis process are the lumbosacral region MRI, X-ray, and urodynamic testing [12, 13, 27, 28].

Magnetic resonance imaging is the imaging modality of preference for diagnosing TFTS, which is used mainly to evaluate the conus medullaris' level, assess the filum terminale's thickness, and look for the presence of fatty filum. The level of the conus medullaris is determined using sagittal T1 and T2 weighted images. A suggestive diagnosis might come in a picture of conus medullaris that is low-lying is often strongly linked to a TFTS, however, the diagnosis of TFTS is not excluded by a normal position of the conus medullaris. Axial T1 scans are used to determine the filum terminale diameter and to detect the fatty filum. Normally, the filum terminale diameter at the L5-S1 level disk space is equal to or less than 2 mm. Findings more than 2 mm are considered abnormally large. The hypertonic autonomous bladder is the most common finding in urodynamic studies. Most patients present with an incomplete neurogenic bladder [12, 13, 27–29].

17.4 Management

17.4.1 Preoperative Considerations

One of the treatment options for tight filum terminale is surgical spinal cord untethering via the filum terminale sectioning with the aim of relieving the lower cord tension [9, 15, 27, 30, 31]. On the other hand, the TFTS conservative management is directed toward managing and easing the symptoms, including muscle relaxants, analgesia, physical therapy, and avoidance of vigorous exercises [31]. After reviewing pieces of the literature, most of the articles stated that indications for the untethering surgery are controversial, Selçuki et al. determined that the indications for filum terminale sectioning are (a) Urinary incontinence and (b) hyper-reflexive contractions with hypertonic bladder dysfunction in urodynamic studies [32]. When untethering surgery is indicated, open surgery has good outcomes postoperatively but holds a risk of re-tethering due to tissue trauma and scar formation [33]. So, the neurosurgeon started to move toward the least detrimental procedures like the flavectomy approach to the filum terminale during sectioning, and the endoscopic sectioning of the tight filum terminale with neuromonitoring appeared to be a safe technique that reduces the hospitality and the risk of peri-operational bleeding [32, 33]. A benefit from filum terminale sectioning in TFTS was reported in several studies [9, 15, 27, 30, 32, 34]. Surgical untethering might relieve symptoms and prevent further neurological deterioration [9]. The results of a prospective study on 13 patients with Tight Filum Terminale aged between 5 and 17 years who had normal level conus medullaris demonstrated that about 70% of these patients have benefited from the surgical intervention [32]. This study revealed that none of the patient's age, the presence of Urinary Tract Infection (UTI), the status of toilet training, or the duration of symptoms have affected the surgical outcomes in the patients included in this study [32]. The successful selection of patients and identification of surgical candidates seem to be very crucial to achieve better surgical outcomes [9, 32].

To be able to select suitable candidates for surgery, one should know the relationship between the clinical presentation of the tight filum terminale syndrome and the outcomes of the untethering surgery [9]. In 2009, a retrospective cohort study was carried out to evaluate the preoperative characteristics that may correlate with surgical outcomes following untethering surgery for pediatric patients with tight filum terminale syndrome. This study showed that the patients who presented with symptoms and clinical findings in two or more categories of symptoms (neurologic, urologic, dermatologic, and orthopedic) were more inclined to improve following the untethering surgery than those who presented with symptoms and clinical findings in only one category [9]. But this topic needs to be investigated more, as other preoperative features (if any) need to be identified to ease the selection of surgical candidates in the future.

17.4.2 Intraoperative Management and Procedure

In open untethering surgeries for tight filum terminale syndrome, which is operated under general anesthesia (GA) and after antibiotics administration, the surgeons put the patient in a prone position, placing electrodes for intraoperative electrophysiological monitoring, including an electrode to monitor the electrophysiology of the anal sphincter. The motor evoked potentials (MEPs) and somatosensory evoked potentials (SSEPs) and should be monitored for all the patients. The incision is opened from below the level of L5 to the mid-level of the sacrum then the surgeons carry out an L5 Laminotomy to access the filum terminale. Once the surgeons reach and identify the filum terminale, they should make sure that the filum terminale is free from nerve roots circumferentially before transecting the filum terminale [13, 35].

17.4.3 Postoperative Management

Traditionally, in the postoperative period, the patients who underwent untethering surgery for tight filum terminale were kept in a horizontal decubitus position for 24–72 h [15, 36–40]. The aim of keeping the patients in this position was to prevent the leakage of the Cerebrospinal fluid (CSF) after the surgery [36, 37]. But the optimal period that the patients should be kept in the horizontal position and whether keeping patients in this position actually prevents the leakage of the Cerebrospinal Fluid (CSF) was not known [37]. However, the results of a retrospective cohort study that was conducted on patients who underwent the untethering surgery for tight filum terminale syndrome in Tokyo between 2012 and 2016 suggest that it is not necessary to maintain patients in the horizontal decubitus position following the sectioning of a tight filum terminale in order to prevent CSF leaking [37]. Careful wound management, dressing, and cleaning are necessary. Obtaining Magnetic Resonance Imaging (MRI) for the spine 1 to 2 weeks postoperatively is required for the follow-up of the patients [37].

17.5 Complications

In this paragraph, we are highlighting the complications of surgical untethering, not the disease itself, as the clinical manifestations of the disease are described in the diagnosis section. It was found that tight filum terminale untethering has a 12% total complication rate. The most frequent complications are (a) leakage of CSF/pseduomeningocele, (b) re-tethering, (c) and infection of the surgical wound with rates of 5.9%, 5%, and 4%, respectively [13, 37]. Regarding re-tethering, arachnoid adhesion is the most common cause of it. It may happen many years after the first untethering procedure. Patients with frequent inflammations of the arachnoid, a high conus medullaris, and advanced age are the most probable causes for developing this complication soon after the first untethering surgery [13].

17.6 Prognosis and Outcomes

Many of the reviewed articles showed that the overall outcome of the untethering surgery of the tight filum terminale syndrome is favorable, especially in symptomatic patients with clinical abnormalities in multiple categories of symptoms [9, 13,

15, 27, 30, 32, 34, 35]. After surgical untethering of the filum terminale for patients with TFTS, it was shown that symptomatic pediatric patients had better outcomes than adult patients. Pediatric patients with sensory and motor symptoms show a kind of stabilization in 90%–100% of cases and improvement in 50%–80% of cases. Alleviation of pain was shown in 80%–100% of cases, while patients with scoliosis improved by 37% and stabilized by 63%–87%. Furthermore, 37% of spastic patients improved. Patients with urologic symptoms respond to the untethering procedure 94% of the time, with 43% to 87% of patients improving. For adults, it was found that adult patients with sensorimotor dysfunction improved at similar rates as pediatric patients. On the other hand, adult patients with urologic symptoms showed an improvement in only 33% of patients postoperatively. In occult TFTS patients, the overall improvement is 73%–88% of patients. Patients with urodynamic problems preoperatively showed a 42% improvement after the surgery, while patients who had many systematic signs and symptoms improved 88% of the time [13, 35].

Multiple Choice Questions

1. **Tight filum terminale syndrome is:**

   (a) A general term used to describe abnormally structured filum terminale with loss of its elasticity.
   (b) A subtype of primary tethered cord syndrome caused by shortened or inelastic filum terminale.
   (c) A synonym for tethered cord syndrome.
   (d) A syndrome caused by a filum terminale that is less than 0.4 mm in diameter.

2. **All of the following may be causes of secondary Tethered cord syndrome (TCS), except:**

   (a) Myelomeningocele.
   (b) Lipoma.
   (c) Tight filum terminale.
   (d) Spinal trauma.

3. **Which of the following is not true regarding the lower or distal part of the filum terminale?**

   (a) The mean diameter of the distal part of the filum terminale is about 1.36 mm.
   (b) It is also called filum terminale externum or the coccygeal ligament.
   (c) It is roughly 5 cm long and is earmarked to the dura mater.
   (d) It is the part of the filum terminale that attaches to the dorsal part of the coccyx.

4. **Which of the following is the main factor that plays the key role in the pathophysiology of the *Tight Filum Terminale Syndrome*?**

   (a) Stretching of the lumbosacral spinal nerve roots.
   (b) Traction of the lumbosacral cord especially at the conus medullaris.

(c) Inelasticity of the filum terminale due to apoptosis, tissue necrosis, and fatty infiltration.
(d) Impaired oxidative metabolism in the lumbosacral cord.

5. **Which of the following best explains the musculoskeletal deformities that may occur as a consequence of the Tethered cord syndrome in some patients?**

(a) In response to intramedullary tension, a functional adaptation of the paravertebral muscles occurs to change the curvature of the spinal column in an attempt to minimize the intramedullary tension.
(b) Some of the patients with secondary forms of Tethered cord syndrome (TCS) presented with other associated congenital anomalies of the spine and the spinal cord.
(c) Loss of motor function of the paravertebral muscles causes exaggerated scoliosis of the lumbosacral spine.
(d) All of the above.

6. **Regarding the management of tight filum terminale, we can conclude that:**

(a) Conservative management is superior to surgical management.
(b) Patients with clinical abnormalities in multiple categories of symptoms are more likely to benefit from tight filum terminale sectioning than those with clinical abnormalities in one category of symptoms.
(c) The status of toilet training and the duration of symptoms affect the surgical outcomes in patients with tight filum terminale syndrome.
(d) The endoscopic approach to filum terminale sectioning holds a risk of re-tethering due to massive tissue damage and scar formation.

7. **To prevent the leakage of the Cerebrospinal Fluid after the untethering surgery, the patient should be kept in a horizontal decubitus position for:**

(a) 24 h.
(b) 48 h.
(c) 72 h.
(d) Keeping the patient in a horizontal decubitus position doesn't seem to prevent CSF leakage.

8. **The most frequent complication(s) after untethering surgery for *tight filum terminale syndrome is*:**

(a) Wound infection.
(b) CSF leakage.
(c) Re-tethering.
(d) Arachnoid adhesion.

9. **The most common finding in urodynamic studies in *TFT syndrome* is:**

(a) Neurogenic Bladder.
(b) Hypertonic autonomous bladder.

(c) Flaccid Bladder.
(d) Overactive Bladder.

10. **One of the following imaging modalities are not used specifically for the diagnosis of TFTS:**

(a) Magnetic Resonance Imaging (MRI).
(b) Computed Tomography (CT scan).
(c) Urodynamic Studies.
(d) Plain X-ray.

Answers and Explanations

1. ***The answer is (b)*** Tight Filum Terminale Syndrome is a subtype of Tethered Cord Syndrome (TCS) that is caused by tight and inelastic filum terminale.
2. ***The answer is (c)*** Abnormal tissues attachment is the main pathological factor in primary TCS, like tight filum terminale. Myelomeningocele, lipoma, and spinal trauma are among the causes of secondary TCS.
3. ***The answer is (a)*** The lower or distal part of the filum terminale also known as the coccygeal ligament or the filum terminale externum is nearly 5 cm long and is devoted to the dura mater. The mean diameter of the lower component of the filum terminale is 1 mm or less.
4. ***The answer is (c)*** The tight filum terminale likely results from deviant involution in the form of apoptosis and/or necrosis of the fibers that form the filum terminale, followed by fibrosis and fatty infiltration of the filum, leading to an inelastic filum terminale that causes the lower spinal cord tension.
5. ***The answer is (a)*** As a result of intramedullary tension brought on by cord traction or tethering, the paravertebral muscles adjust reflexively (functionally) to change the curvature of the spinal column, allowing the spinal cord to travel through the spinal column for a shorter distance and reducing intramedullary tension. This results in musculoskeletal abnormalities including scoliosis, high-arched feet, excessive lumbosacral lordosis, and hammer toes.
6. ***The answer is (b)*** According to studies, patients presenting with clinical manifestations of multiple categories are more likely to benefit from the untethering surgery than the patients presenting with clinical manifestations of one category only.
7. ***The answer is (d)*** Recent studies showed that it is not necessary to maintain patients in the horizontal decubitus position following the sectioning of a tight filum terminale in order to prevent CSF leaking.
8. ***The answer is (b)*** The rate of CSF leakage after untethering surgery for TFTS is about 5.9%, making it as the most common complication after the untethering surgery.
9. ***The answer is (b)*** The hypertonic autonomous bladder is the most common finding in urodynamic studies of patients with TFTS. Most patients present with an incomplete neurogenic bladder.
10. ***The answer is (d)*** Plain X-rays are used in scoliotic deformity evaluation as part of the preoperative planning and assessment and are not used specifically for the diagnosis of TFTS.

References

1. Choi BH, Kim RC, Suzuki M, Choe W. The ventriculus terminalis and filum terminale of the human spinal cord. Hum Pathol. 1992;23(8):916–20.
2. Barkovich J, Raybaud C. Congenital anomalies of the spine. In: Schwartz ES, Barkovich AJ, editors. Pediatric neuroimaging. 6th ed. Lippincott Williams & Wilkins; 2019.
3. Saker E, Henry BM, Tomaszewski KA, Loukas M, Iwanaga J, Oskouian RJ, et al. The filum terminale internum and externum: a comprehensive review. J Clin Neurosci. 2017;40:6–13.
4. Cramer G, Darby S. Basic and clinical anatomy of the spine, spinal cord, and ANS. 2nd ed. Elsevier Health Sciences; 2005.
5. Jiang Q, Tao B, Gao G, Sun M, Wang H, Li J, et al. Filum terminale: a comprehensive review with anatomical, pathological, and surgical considerations. World Neurosurg. 2022;(164):167–76.
6. Nasr AY, Hussein AM, Zaghloul SA. Morphometric parameters and histological study of the filum terminale of adult human cadavers and magnetic resonance images. Folia Morphologica (Poland). 2018;77(4)
7. Gray H. In: Standring S, editor. Gray's anatomy: the anatomical basis of clinical practice. 39th ed. Elsevier Churchill Livingstone; 2005.
8. Sato T, Eguchi Y, Enomoto K, Murata Y. Treating difficult-to-diagnose tight filum terminale: our experience with four patients. BMJ Case Rep. 2021;14(2)
9. Fabiano AJ, Khan MF, Rozzelle CJ, Li V. Preoperative predictors for improvement after surgical untethering in occult tight filum terminale syndrome. Pediatr Neurosurg. 2009;45(4):256–61.
10. Ramina R, Pires de Aguiar P, Tatagiba M. Primary tethered cord syndrome. In: Rosahl S, editor. Samii's essentials in neurosurgery. 2nd ed. Springer. p. 449–60.
11. Kiechl S, Kronenberg MF, Marosi M, Birbamer GG, Saltuari L. Tethered cord syndrome as cause of spinal cord dysfunction [20]. Lancet. 1996;348:342–3.
12. Raghavan N, Barkovich AJ, Edwards M, Norman D. MR imaging in the tethered spinal cord syndrome. Am J Roentgenol. 1989;152(4):843–52.
13. Cohen A. Tight filum terminale. In: Wilson T, Muraszko K, editors. Pediatric neurosurgery: tricks of the trade. Thieme Medical Publishers; 2016.
14. Khoury AE, Hendrick EB, McLorie GA, Kulkarni A, Churchill BM. Occult spinal dysraphism: clinical and urodynamic outcome after division of the filum terminale. J Urol. 1990;144:426–8.
15. Wehby MC, O'Hollaren PS, Abtin K, Hume JL, Richards BJ. Occult tight filum terminale syndrome: results of surgical untethering. Pediatr Neurosurg. 2004;40:51–7.
16. Steinbok P, MacNeily AE. Section of the terminal filum for occult tethered cord syndrome: toward a scientific answer. Neurosurg Focus. 2007;23:1–4.
17. Zalatimo O. Tethered spinal cord syndrome [Internet]. American Association of Neurological Surgeons. [cited 2022 Oct 17].. Available from: https://www.aans.org/patients/neurosurgical-conditions-and-treatments/tethered-spinal-cord-syndrome
18. Filippidis AS, Kalani MY, Theodore N, Rekate HL. Spinal cord traction, vascular compromise, hypoxia, and metabolic derangements in the pathophysiology of tethered cord syndrome. Neurosurg Focus. 2010;29(1):E9.
19. Doczi T, Szerdahelyi P, Gulya K, Kiss J. Brain water accumulation after the central administration of vasopressin. Neurosurgery. 1982;11(3):402–7.
20. Bao N, Chen ZH, Gu S, Chen QM, Jin HM, Shi CR. Tight filum terminale syndrome in children: analysis based on positioning of the conus and absence or presence of lumbosacral lipoma. Childs Nerv Syst. 2007;23(10):1129–34.
21. Hendson G, Dunham C, Steinbok P. Histopathology of the filum terminale in children with and without tethered cord syndrome with attention to the elastic tissue within the filum. Childs Nerv Syst. 2016;32(9):1683–92.
22. Barutcuoglu M, Selcuki M, Selcuki D, Umur S, Mete M, Gurgen SG, et al. Cutting filum terminale is very important in split cord malformation cases to achieve total release. Childs Nerv Syst. 2015;31(3):425–32.

23. Yamada S, Won DJ, Pezeshkpour G, Yamada BS, Yamada SM, Siddiqi J, et al. Pathophysiology of tethered cord syndrome and similar complex disorders. Neurosurg Focus. 2007;23:1–10.
24. Yamada S, Won DJ, Yamada SM. Pathophysiology of tethered cord syndrome: correlation with symptomatology. Neurosurg Focus. 2004;16:1–5.
25. Kwon B, Kim DH, Vaccaro AR. The pathophysiology of tethered cord syndrome: ischemia or apoptosis? Semin Spine Surg. 2005;17(1):8–12.
26. Bierbrauer K, Kuntz C, Ostling L. Fatty filum terminale: part I—diagnosis. Contemp Neurosurg. 2012;34(20):1–5.
27. Komagata M, Endo K, Nishiyama M, Ikegami H, Imakiire A. Management of tight filum terminale. Minim Invasive Neurosurg. 2004;47:49–53.
28. Elmesallamy W, AbdAlwanis A, Mohamed S. Tethered cord syndrome: surgical outcome of 43 cases and review of literatures. Egypt J Neurosurg. 2019;34(1)
29. Bierbrauer K, Kuntz C, Ostling L. Fatty filum terminale: part I—diagnosis. Contemp Neurosurg [Internet]. 2012;34(20) Available from: http://journals.lww.com/contempneurosurg/Abstract/2012/10150/Fatty_Filum_Terminale___Part_I_Diagnosis.1.aspx
30. Selçuki M, Ünlü A, Uğur HÇ, Soygür T, Arikan N, Selçuki D. Patients with urinary incontinence often benefit from surgical detethering of tight filum terminale. Childs Nerv Syst. 2000;16(3):150–4.
31. Lew SM, Kothbauer KF. Tethered cord syndrome: an updated review. Pediatr Neurosurg. 2007;43:236–48.
32. Selçuki M, Coşkun K. Management of tight filum terminale syndrome: with special emphasis on normal level conus medullaris (NLCM). Surg Neurol. 1998;50(4):318–22.
33. Okay O, Dalgic A, Yildirim AE, Ucer M, Uckun O, Baydin S, et al. Endoscopic untethering of tight filum terminale: an operative technique. Turk Neurosurg. 2021;31(1)
34. Metcalfe PD, Luerssen TG, King SJ, Kaefer M, Meldrum KK, Cain MP, et al. Treatment of the occult tethered spinal cord for neuropathic bladder: results of sectioning the filum Terminale. J Urol. 2006;176(4 SUPPL):1826–30.
35. Bierbrauer K, Kuntz C, Ostling L. Fatty filum Terminale: part II — surgical technique and outcomes. Contemp Neurosurg. 2012;34(21)
36. Chern JJ, Tubbs RS, Patel AJ, Gordon AS, Bandt SK, Smyth MD, et al. Preventing cerebrospinal fluid leak following transection of a tight filum terminale: clinical article. J Neurosurg Pediatr. 2011;8(1):35–8.
37. Kanematsu R, Hirokawa D, Usami K, Ogiwara H. Is the postoperative horizontal decubitus position following transection of a tight filum Terminale in pediatric patients necessary?-a retrospective cohort study. Neurol Med Chir (Tokyo). 2020;60:252–5.
38. Ogiwara H, Joko M, Takado M, Uematsu K, Kameda M, Sasaki N, et al. Duration of the horizontal decubitus position for prevention of cerebrospinal fluid leakage following transection of a tight filum terminale. J Neurosurg Pediatr. 2015;15(5):461–4.
39. Ogiwara H, Morota N, Joko M. Duration of horizontal decubitus after section of a tight filum terminale as a means to prevent cerebrospinal fluid leakage. Surg Neurol Int. 2012;3(1):113.
40. Chern JJ, Dauser RC, Whitehead WE, Curry DJ, Luerssen TG, Jea A. The effect of tethered cord release on coronal spinal balance in tight filum terminale. Spine. 2011;36:E944–9.

Chapter 18
Abnormally Elongated Spinal Cord

Ahmed Hassan A. Rady and Mohammedbaqer Ali Al-Ghuraibawi

Test your learning and check your understanding of this book's contents: use the "Springer Nature Flashcards" app to access questions using ▶ https://sn.pub/QCsfpd.
To use the app, please follow the instructions in Chap. 1

18.1 Overview

A neurological spinal cord syndrome occurs when spinal cord tissue attachments limit the movement of the spinal cord within the spinal canal, causing abnormal elongation of the cord [1]. This is associated with spina bifida, which is a congenital defect of the spinal cord. About 20–50% of spina bifida children require surgical treatment to untether the spinal cord [2].

Spina bifida is a congenital disorder where the spinal cord of the child doesn't develop accurately in the uterus creating a gap in the spine, and this type of neurological defect occurs when the structure that eventually develops into the child's central nervous system, called the neural tube doesn't develop or close properly resulting in defects in the spinal cord and vertebrae [3, 4]. Normally the neural tube starts to form during early pregnancy and closes around 4 weeks after conception [5, 6].

A. H. A. Rady (✉)
Faculty of Medicine, Ain Shams University, Cairo, Egypt

M. A. Al-Ghuraibawi
Faculty of Medicine, University of Warith Al-Anbiyaa, Karbala, Iraq

K. F. AlAli, H. T. Hashim (eds.), *Congenital Spine Malformations*,
https://doi.org/10.1007/978-3-031-59031-3_18

Epidemiology: About 1427 babies annually are born with spinal bifida in the United States. People, cultures, or countries related to Spain, or Spanish language (Hispanic) women have a higher rate of having a child with spina bifida, otherwise, non-Hispanic women [7–10].

Nearly 3.8 each of 10,000 live births in Hispanics are born with spina bifida, 2.7 each of 10,000 in non-Hispanic black women, and 3.09 each of 10,000 births in non-Hispanic white women [8, 9, 11].

18.2 Types of Spina Bifida

Spina bifida is of several types, this condition may present in various forms, including open spina bifida (spina bifida cystica, myelomeningocele, and meningocele), closed spina bifida (lipo-myelomeningocele, and diastematomyelia) [12, 13].

Open spina bifida (spina bifida cystica): characterized by a visible sac or cyst on the back of the patient, like a large blister [14, 15].

Myelomeningocele (Meningomyelocele): the commonest among all types of cystic spinal bifida, it is characterized by that the cyst contains nerves and parts from the spinal cord in addition to tissue and cerebrospinal fluid (CSF) [16]. During pregnancy, the development of the spinal cord is damaged by fluid in the uterus, which leads to this defect. This damage results almost always in paralysis and sensation loss, furthermore, the nerves to and from the cord are impacted [17, 18–20].

Meningocele: less common than other cystic types of spina bifida and usually causes less severe development impairment than other types. It is characterized by the sac doesn't contain spinal tissue, but it contains meninges and cerebrospinal fluid (CSF).

Closed spina bifida: this condition of spinal disorder is characterized by the skin covering the sac, unlike open spina bifida where the skin doesn't cover and the cyst is exposed [21].

Spina bifida occulta (SBO): when there is one or more than one vertebrae are not closed completely. This form of spina bifida is covered by skin and it includes many specific conditions such as lipo-myelomeningocele, tethered cord, or diastematomyelia. Each specific type requires a different approach to treatment, so it is very important to distinguish between each type [22, 23].

SBO is not a rare condition, there are around 5-–10 million people who may have one or more open vertebrae or incompletely closed vertebrae, typically around the age of 16–18 bone growth is complete, which means children have a higher rate of incidence compared with adults. Most people with spina bifida occulta are not aware of it, it could be discovered by accident while looking for other diseases for any other cause, such as doing an MRI for any purpose. So people with SBO would be asymptomatic or with symptoms [24, 25].

SBO can occur anywhere along the spine but is most commonly at the level of L5\S1. Some patients with SBO may experience pain and nerve)defects due to decreased spinal stability, keeping in mind that SBO can be associated with other spinal bone conditions including pars defect (a small hairline fracture of part of the vertebrae), spondylosis (spine arthritis), and spondylolisthesis (A slips of the vertebral body causing radicular or mechanical symptoms or pain). For some people's presentation of SBO is low back pain. We should investigate properly to detect the underlying cause [26]. If the patient is diagnosed with SBO with no symptoms, the patient can keep moving in usual activities with follow-up [27–29].

Closed spinal dysraphism can lead to various conditions that can significantly impact an individual's life and abilities, While the term "spina bifida occulta" is sometimes used to refer to other skin-covered lesions such as lipo-myelomeningocele and diastematomyelia, it is more beneficial to differentiate between these conditions and uncomplicated gaps in the vertebrae from a clinical perspective [30, 31].

Individuals with closed spinal dysraphism may experience nerve and spinal cord complications as opposed to solely gaps in the vertebrae [32]. This condition may be accompanied by a fatty lump embedded in the spinal column, known as lipomyelomeningocele, or a bone fragment dividing the spinal cord, known as diastematomyelia. Physical indications on the back may include a lump, a hemangioma, or naevus (strawberry birthmark), a tuft of hair resembling head hair instead of down back hair, or a deep dimple or sinus above the cleft of the gluteal region [33]. It is important to understand that small indentations in the gluteal region crease are quite common and typically unrelated to spinal dysraphism [34]. Spina bifida occulta occurs when nerves and spinal tissue become trapped, entangled in fatty masses, or caught up in abnormal bone structures, which can restrict movement of the spine within the spinal column [35]. Fortunately, the skin covering the spinal cord provides a protective barrier against the potentially harmful effects of amniotic fluid exposure in myelomeningocele (open spina bifida), while symptoms may occasionally arise at birth, they more commonly emerge during periods of rapid growth in childhood or middle age, these symptoms may include back pain, inward-turning feet (Talipes), growing pain, weakness, fatigue, or pain while walking, leg)and foot cramps, calf muscle atrophy, numbness or loss of sensation in the feet, as well as bladder and\or bowel issues [36].

Lipomyelomeningocoele: it is known as a congenital spinal cord disorder mainly is caused by the entanglement of a benign fatty tumor with part of the spinal cord and nerves. Lip-myelomeningocele could develop during the period of early stages of pregnancy as a result of a failure of the neural tube closure, and its exact cause is still uncertain [37]. The fatty tissue attaches to the spinal cord when the layer of the skin detaches from the neural tissue early, which leads to leaving the spina bifida gap. This gap could prevent the spinal bones from completely closing, resulting in a skin-covered lump on the baby's back at birth, which can vary in size, shape, and location. Most majority of those affected by lipomyelomeningocele exhibit markers at the site of the lesion such as fatty lumps, deep dimples, or birthmarks, which is an indication for the presentation of this condition [38].

On the other hand, lipo-myelomeningocele represents nearly 15% of all cases of spina bifida, it can not be detectable during the antenatal mid-term ultrasound, which leads to identify significant fetal abnormalities [39]. In spina bifida Aperta (open spina bifida), the appearance of the skull bones and cerebellum exhibit distinct signs that lead the sonographer to look for tiny changes in the spine [40]. However, in lipomyelomeningocele, the brain and skull usually may appear normal, resulting in the changes in the spine going unremarkable [41, 42]. Therefore, the diagnosis is generally made after birth, based mainly on physical examination and imaging tests, including magnetic resonance imaging (MRI), which can provide detailed results about the status of the spinal cord and the surrounding structures [43].

Since lipomyelomeningocele is covered by the skin, there is no need for back closure surgery at birth, and it usually does not affect brain development. Around 5% of those affected by the condition may experience other complications that can impact their quality of life and necessitate medical intervention [44]. One of the most common complications is Tethered cord syndrome, which occurs when the spinal cord and nerves become trapped within the fatty lump, leading to spinal nerve problems such as back pain, leg weakness, numbness, or bladder and bowel dysfunction [45]. Tethered cord syndrome can cause neurological damage if left untreated [46].

Hydrocephalus is another potential complication of lipomyelomeningocele, which characterized by a massive accumulation of cerebrospinal fluid (CSF) in the brain ventricles, leading to increased pressure and swelling. Hydrocephalus can occur if the fatty lump compresses the cerebral aqueduct, a narrow channel that connects the third and fourth ventricles in the brain [47]. Hydrocephalus can be represented by several symptoms as headaches, nausea, vomiting, seizures, vision problems, and developmental delays if not treated. Treatment for hydrocephalus usually involves the insertion of a shunt, a flexible tube that drains the excess fluid from the brain to another part of the body where it can be absorbed [48].

Lipomyelomeningocoele usually affects the bladder and bowel, resulting in difficulties with potty training, frequency or urgency of passing urine, a poor, dribbling stream of urine in boys, or urine infections [49]. These symptoms can be due to neurogenic bladder, a condition in which the nerves that control the bladder and the sphincter muscles are difunctionally affected. Urinary incontinence can occur, urinary retention, or urinary tract infections (UTIs), which can be painful and potentially harmful. Children with nerve conditions affecting their bladders must have their bladder function checked regularly by a urologist to prevent long-term complications such as kidney damage or bladder stones [50].

If necessary, lipomyelomeningocele is typically treated by surgery to release the nerves from within the fatty lump. Neurosurgeons differ in their approaches to surgery by the time of surgery. Scar tissue from the surgery can cause further tethering, and waiting may result in fewer untethering operations over a person's lifetime. Sometimes, the nerves are entangled in the fatty lump, making it impossible to free all the nerves or remove all the fat. In such cases, the surgery's goal is to improve symptoms and prevent further damage rather than cure the condition [51]. Regular monitoring of the condition is critical, and any changes should be reported to your neurosurgeon immediately to prevent complications and optimize the long-term outcome [52].

Diastematomyelia: is a congenital disorder that hampers the development of the spinal cord. Diastematomyelia is characterized by a split in the spinal cord into two longitudinal halves, usually in the lumbar region [53–55]. The split can occur due to an additional piece of bone or a band of fibrous tissue, which may also lead to diplomyelia [56]. The presence of the extra bone or tissue can cause the spinal cord to become tethered, which in turn can lead to a range of symptoms such as back pain, muscle weakness, and dysfunction of the bowel or bladder. Treatment for diastematomyelia is detethering, which includes the removal of the additional bone or tissue aiming to spinal cord free. However, individuals without additional bone or tissue may only experience symptoms if the cord becomes tethered [57, 58]. In some cases, diastematomyelia may coexist with lipomyelomeningocele, a type of neural tube defect marked by the spinal cord and its covering protruding through a defect in the vertebral column [59].

Symptoms: Spina bifida is a very complex medical condition that is characterized by the not-so-going development of the spinal cord. The condition can cause a variety of symptoms that can have a significant impact on the affected individual's life. These symptoms can include issues with movement, bladder and bowel control problems, and complications associated with the accumulation of excess fluid in the brain, which is also known as hydrocephalus [60].

The severity of the symptoms experienced by individuals with spina bifida can vary widely depending on the location of the spinal cord gap. If the gap is present higher up the spine, it is more likely to result in paralysis of the legs and mobility difficulties. In contrast, if the gap is located in the middle or at the base of the spine, it may only cause issues related to continence [61].

Most of the children diagnosed with spina bifida experience weakness or paralysis of the lower limbs. This can make it challenging for them to walk, and they may require ankle support or crutches to assist with their mobility [62].

Paralysis can lead to other associated complications, such as muscle weakness. Misshapen bones, fractures of bones, and dislocated or deformed joints can result, as well as abnormal spinal development, which can lead to scoliosis [63].

Bladder problems are a common issue for individuals with spina bifida due to the nerves responsible for bladder control not forming properly [64]. This can lead to several complications, including urinary incontinence, kidney stones, urinary tract infections (UTIs), kidney scarring, and hydronephrosis, which is when one or both kidneys become swollen due to a buildup of urine. To prevent any complications, it is crucial to monitor the bladder and kidneys regularly, with ultrasound scans and volume measurement tests used to check the bladder's volume and the pressure inside it.

Bowel problems can also be a common issue for individuals with spina bifida due to the nerves that control the bowel and sphincter muscles, which are responsible for keeping feces in the bowel [65, 66]. This can result in limited or no control over the sphincter muscles and bowel incontinence. As a result, individuals with spina bifida often experience constipation followed by episodes of diarrhea or soiling [67].

Spina bifida is a birth defect that affects the spinal cord and can lead to a wide range of complications. One of the most significant complications is the development of hydrocephalus, which is the accumulation of massive fluid in the brain. Hydrocephalus can lead to brain damage, resulting in more complications [68, 69].

patients with spina bifida and hydrocephalus may have average IQ levels, but some may struggle with learning difficulties, such as short attention spans, problem-solving, reading, and understanding fast conversations between groups. They may also experience difficulties in organizing activities or making detailed plans, as well as problems with visual and physical coordination, As in tying shoelaces or fastening buttons [70].

Type 2 Arnold-Chiari malformation meant by that In some infants with spina bifida, the brain's lower parts are displaced downwards towards the spinal cord. This condition is related to the development of hydrocephalus. Hydrocephalus can cause additional symptoms soon after birth, such as seizures, irritability, drowsiness, poor feeding, and vomiting [71, 72].

Early detection of hydrocephalus is very important to start initial treatment, also to prevent more unwanted complications.

Spina bifida is a condition that can lead to various problems, including skin problems. Decreasing sensation ability may lead to infection and ulcers. Therefore, it's important to check the skin regularly for any signs of injury. People with spina bifida may develop an allergy to latex.

18.3 Causes

Having a deficiency of folic acid during pregnancy is a crucial factor that can increase the likelihood of giving birth to a child with spina bifida. Folic acid (vitamin B9) is found naturally in some foods. Folic acid supplements can be used. It is suggested that taking folic acid supplements before and during pregnancy may prevent up to 7 out of 10 cases of neural tube defects, such as spina bifida. Although it is not clear how folic acid helps prevent spina bifida, it is believed that folic acid is necessary for important biochemical reactions in the body [73].

Family history: Having a family member with a neural tube defect, such as spina bifida, increases your chances of having a baby with spina bifida. If you've previously had a child with spina bifida, your chance of having other children with the condition is increased. If you have a family history of spina bifida, you must take high-dose folic acid, prescribed by a GP before you become pregnant, and for at least the first 12 weeks of pregnancy [74].

Medication: Taking certain medications during pregnancy has been associated with an increased risk of having a baby with spina bifida. *Valproate* and *carbamazepine* that are used to treat epilepsy and some mental health conditions such as bipolar disorder, and have been linked to spina bifida. While doctors will attempt to avoid prescribing these medicines if there is a possibility of becoming pregnant while taking them, they may still be required if alternative treatments are ineffective. If you need to take one of these medicines and are not trying to conceive, it is recommended that you use a reliable form of contraception. If you are planning to have a baby and need to take one of these medicines, inform your doctor. They may be able to lower the dosage and prescribe folic acid supplements at a higher than normal dose, to minimize the risk of issues. If you are uncertain if a medicine could affect your pregnancy, it is always best to consult with your doctor, midwife, or pharmacist before taking it. It is never recommended to stop taking any prescribed medication unless advised to do so by a healthcare professional responsible for your care.

Genetic: Spina bifida can rarely occur alongside genetic conditions such as *Patau's syndrome*, *Edwards' syndrome,* or *Down's syndrome* in babies. If your baby is diagnosed with spina bifida and there is a possibility of them having one of these syndromes, your healthcare provider may suggest diagnostic tests like amniocentesis or chorionic villus sampling. These tests can precisely determine whether your baby has any of these genetic conditions [73].

Another factors are: - Obesity: Women who have a body mass index of 30 or more are at a higher risk of having a baby with spina bifida.

- Women with diabetes may also have an increased risk of having a child with spina bifida.

Detecting Spina Bifida: Spina bifida is typically identified during the mid-pregnancy anomaly scan, which is offered to all pregnant women from 18 to 21 weeks of pregnancy. Diagnosis and Treatment: If the tests confirm that the baby has spina bifida, the implications will be discussed with the parents. This discussion will include possible problems associated with the condition, the treatment and support the baby may need if the parents decide to continue with the pregnancy, and the options available if they decide to terminate the pregnancy. Post-birth Tests: After the baby is born, several tests may be carried out to find out the severity of the condition and decide which treatment options are best. These tests may include monitoring the baby's head growth and carrying out a brain scan, using an ultrasound scan, CT scan, or MRI scan to check for hydrocephalus (excess fluid on the brain), ultrasound scans of the bladder and kidneys to check whether the baby stores pee normally, and an assessment of the baby's movements to check for paralysis. Surgery: Surgery to repair the spine will usually be recommended soon after the baby is born.

Treatment: If your child has been diagnosed with spina bifida of any type, they will be referred to a specialist team that will be responsible for their care. A care plan may be developed to address your child's needs and any issues they may be facing. As your child grows older, the care plan will be reviewed and modified to account for changes in their needs and circumstances. There are several different treatments available to address the various issues that spina bifida can cause [75].

Surgery: When babies are born with spina bifida, there is a possibility that nerves and membranes may protrude through an opening in their spine, forming a sac. This can lead to nerve damage and serious infections, so it's necessary to have surgery to repair the spine within 48 h of birth. During the surgery, the surgeon will place the spinal cord, tissues, and nerves back into the correct position. The gap in the spine will be closed, and the hole will be sealed with muscle and skin. It's important to note that although this operation can repair the defect, it cannot reverse any nerve damage that may have already occurred.

Treating hydrocephalus: Treating hydrocephalus typically requires surgery if a child has an excess of fluid in the brain [74]. During the procedure, a surgeon will implant a thin tube known as a shunt to drain away the excess fluid into another part of the body, mainly the abdomen. The shunt will generally remain in place for the rest of his life. However, further surgery may be necessary if the shunt becomes blocked or infected, or if the child grows and needs a larger shunt.

Physiotherapy plays a crucial role in helping individuals with spina bifida attain maximum independence. The primary objective of physiotherapy is to promote mobility, prevent deformity, and halt further weakening of the leg muscles. This may entail performing daily exercises to maintain leg muscle strength and wearing specialized splints to provide leg support [76].

Occupational therapy is a kind of therapy that can assist individuals in learning how to perform daily activities on their own, thereby increasing their independence.

For individuals who are unable to use their legs, a wheelchair is necessary. Using a manual wheelchair can aid in preserving upper body strength. For those with weak leg muscles, leg braces, splints, and other walking aids can be beneficial.

18.4 Preventing Spina Bifida with Folic Acid

Taking folic acid supplements before and during pregnancy is the most effective way to prevent spina bifida. It is recommended to take a 400 μg folic acid tablet daily while trying to conceive and until the 12th week of pregnancy. It is important to start as soon as you find out you are pregnant If you did not take folic acid before conception. Foods that contain folate such as broccoli, spinach, and chickpeas are also recommended [74].

It is recommended that women who are at a higher risk of giving birth to a child with spina bifida should be prescribed a higher dose (5 mg) of folic acid by their GP. Women who fall into this category include those:

Individuals with a family history of neural tube defects, who have a partner with such history, or who have had a previous pregnancy affected by a neural tube defect, may have an increased risk of having a baby with such a defect [77].

Multiple Choice Questions

1. **All of the following about the treatment of spina bifida are correct except:**

   a. *Occupational therapy* is a kind of therapy that can assist individuals in learning how to perform daily activities on their own.
   b. *Physiotherapy* plays a crucial role in helping individuals with spina bifida attain maximum independence.
   c. Treating hydrocephalus typically does not require surgery if a child has an excess of fluid in the brain.
   d. When bone development is affected, corrective surgery may be required to address issues such as hip dislocation or clubfoot (a deformity of the foot and ankle).
   e. It's important to note that although this operation can repair the defect.

2. **All the following about spina bifida are correct except:**
   a. Most children diagnosed with spina bifida experience some degree of weakness or paralysis in their lower limbs.
   b. Meningomyelocele is the most common among all types of cystic spinal bifida.
   c. Spina bifida can rarely occur alongside genetic conditions such as *Patau's syndrome*, *Edwards' syndrome,* or *Down's syndrome* in babies.
   d. Spina bifida is typically identified during the mid-pregnancy anomaly scan.
   e. MRI is with no benefit in detecting spina bifida.

3. **All the following are true regarding the epidemiology of spina bifida except:**
   a. About 1427 babies annually are born with spinal bifida in the United States.
   b. About 3.09 each of 10,000 births in non-Hispanic white women.
   c. Hispanic women have a lower rate of having a child with spina bifida.
   d. Hispanic women have a higher rate of having a child with spina bifida.
   e. Nearly 3.8 each of 10,000 live births in Hispanics are born with spina bifida.

4. **All of the following statements about the etiology of spina bifida are correct except:**
   a. Having a family member with a neural tube defect, such as spina bifida, increases your chances of having a baby with spina bifida.
   b. *Valproate* and *carbamazepine* are two such medicines with no association with spina bifida.
   c. Spina bifida can rarely occur alongside genetic conditions such as *Patau's syndrome*, *Edwards' syndrome,* or *Down's syndrome* in babies.
   d. Women with diabetes may also have an increased risk of having a child with spina bifida.
   e. Women who have a body mass index (BMI) of 30 or more are at a higher risk of having a baby with spina bifida.

5. **All the following statements about symptoms of spina bifida are true except:**
   a. *Paralysis.*
   b. *Bowel problems.*
   c. *Weakness.*
   d. development of hydrocephalus.
   e. None of the above.

6. **Regarding the prevention of spinal bifida, all the following are correct except:**
   a. Taking folic acid supplements before and during pregnancy is the most effective way to prevent spina bifida.
   b. It is recommended that women who are at a higher risk of giving birth to a child with spina bifida should be prescribed a higher dose (5 mg) of folic acid by their GP.

c. If you did not take folic acid before conception, it is important to start as soon as you find out you are pregnant.
d. It is recommended to take a 400 μg folic acid tablet daily while trying to conceive and until the 12th week of pregnancy.
e. incorporating foods that contain folate such as broccoli, spinach, and chick-peas in your diet is not recommended.

7. **Regarding spina bifida, all the following are correct except:**

   a. If you have a family history of spina bifida, you must take high-dose folic acid, prescribed by a GP before you become pregnant, and for at least the first 12 weeks of pregnancy.
   b. The standard treatment for diastematomyelia is detethering, which includes the removal of the additional bone or tissue aiming to spinal cord free.
   c. A potential complication of lipomyelomeningocele is hydrocephalus.
   d. Closed spina bifida is characterized by skin covering.
   e. Open spina bifida is characterized by covering of the skin.

8. **Spina bifida occulta (SBO) is characterized by all the following except:**

   a. Individuals with closed spinal dysraphism may experience nerve and spinal cord complications as opposed to solely gaps in the vertebrae.
   b. SBO can occur anywhere along the spine but is most commonly at the level of C5.
   c. Patients with SBO can experience weakness, fatigue, or pain while walking, leg and foot cramps, calf muscle atrophy, numbness or loss of sensation in the feet, as well as bladder and bowel issues.
   d. SBO is not a rare condition, there are around 5–10 million people who may have one or more open vertebrae or incompletely closed vertebrae.
   e. Closed spinal dysraphism can lead to various conditions that can significantly impact an individual's life and abilities.

9. **Regarding lipo-myelomeningocele, all the following statements are correct except:**

   a. is a congenital spinal cord disorder caused by the entanglement of a benign fatty tumor with part of the spinal cord and nerves.
   b. represents approximately 75% of the cases of spina bifida.
   c. Hydrocephalus can occur if the fatty lump compresses the cerebral aqueduct.
   d. It is skin-covered.
   e. It is typically treated by surgery to release the nerves from within the fatty lump.

10. **Regarding the management of spina bifida, which of the following statement is incorrect:**

    a. Treating hydrocephalus typically requires surgery if a child has an excess of fluid in the brain.
    b. Spina bifida is typically identified during the mid-pregnancy anomaly scan, which is offered to all pregnant women from 18 to 21 weeks of pregnancy.

c. It is recommended that women who are at a higher risk of giving birth to a child with spina bifida should be prescribed a higher dose (5 mg) of folic acid by their GP.
d. For individuals who are unable to use their legs, a wheelchair is typically necessary.
e. For Patient with a family history of spina bifida, it is not necessary to take folic acid.

References

1. Botto LD, Moore CA, Khoury MJ, Erickson JD. Neural-tube defects. N Engl J Med. 1999;341(20):1509–19.
2. Greene NDE, Copp AJ. Neural tube defects. Annu Rev Neurosci. 2014;37:221–42.
3. Thunem NY, Lowry RB, Tucker BJ, Medd BW. Birth prevalence and recurrence rates of neural tube defects in southern Alberta in 1970-81. CMAJ (Can Med Assoc J). 1988;138(9):819–23.
4. Williams J, Mai CT, Mulinare J, et al. Updated estimates of neural tube defects prevented by mandatory folic acid fortification — United States, 1995–2011. MMWR Morb Mortal Wkly Rep. 2015;64(1):1–5.
5. Copp AJ, Greene NDE. Neural tube defects—disorders of neurulation and related embryonic processes. Wiley Interdiscip Rev Dev Biol. 2013;2(2):213–27.
6. Moore K, Persaud TVN, Torchia M. Before we are born: essentials of embryology and birth defects. 8th ed. Philadelphia: Elsevier; 2011.
7. Nakatsu T, Uwabe C, Shiota K. Neural tube closure in humans initiates at multiple sites: evidence from human embryos and implications for the pathogenesis of neural tube defects. Anat Embryol (Berl). 2000;201(6):455–66.
8. Copp AJ, Brook FA. Does lumbosacral spina bifida arise by failure of neural folding or by defective canalisation? J Med Genet. 1989;26(3):160–6.
9. Morioka T, Hashiguchi K, Mukae N, Sayama T, Sasaki T. Neurosurgical management of patients with lumbosacral myeloschisis. Neurol Med Chir (Tokyo). 2010;50(9):870–6.
10. Northrup H, Volcik KA. Spina bifida and other neural tube defects. Curr Probl Pediatr. 2000;30(10):313–32.
11. Sepulveda W, Wong AE, Sepulveda F, Alcalde JL, Devoto JC, Otayza F. Prenatal diagnosis of spina bifida: from intracranial translucency to intrauterine surgery. Childs Nerv Syst. 2017;33(7):1083–99.
12. Murakami N, Morioka T, Suzuki SO, et al. Clinicopathological findings of limited dorsal myeloschisis associated with spinal lipoma of dorsal-type. Interdiscip Neurosurg. 2020. [Epub ahead of print];21:100781.
13. Meadows JT Jr, Hayes D Jr. Rachischisis totalis without acrania in a newborn male. Pediatr Neurol. 2014;51(1):123–5.
14. Pang D, Zovickian J, Wong ST, Hou YJ, Moes GS. Limited dorsal myeloschisis: a not-so-rare form of primary neurulation defect. Childs Nerv Syst. 2013;29(9):1459–84.
15. Pang D, Zovickian J, Oviedo A, Moes GS. Limited dorsal myeloschisis: a distinctive clinicopathological entity. Neurosurgery. 2010;67(6):1555–80.
16. Morioka T, Suzuki SO, Murakami N, et al. Neurosurgical pathology of limited dorsal myeloschisis. Childs Nerv Syst. 2018;34(2):293–303.
17. Izci Y, Kural C. Limited dorsal myeloschisis with and without type I split cord malformation: report of 3 cases and surgical nuances. Medicine (Kaunas). 2019;55(2):28.
18. Urui S, Oi S. Experimental study of the embryogenesis of open spinal dysraphism. Neurosurg Clin North Am. 1995;6(2):195–202.

19. Dias MS, Walker ML. The embryogenesis of complex dysraphic malformations: a disorder of gastrulation? Pediatr Neurosurg. 1992;18(5–6):229–53.
20. Elgamal EA. Natural history of hydrocephalus in children with spinal open neural tube defect. Surg Neurol Int. 2012;3:112.
21. Cleland. Contribution to the study of spina bifida, encephalocele, and anencephalus. J Anat Physiol. 1883;17(Pt 3):257–92.
22. McLone DG, Knepper PA. The cause of Chiari II malformation: a unified theory. Pediatr Neurosci. 1989;15(1):1–12.
23. Hahn YS. Open myelomeningocele. Neurosurg Clin N Am. 1995;6(2):231–41.
24. Pang D. Surgical complications of open spinal dysraphism. Neurosurg Clin N Am. 1995;6(2):243–57.
25. Babcook CJ. Ultrasound evaluation of prenatal and neonatal spina bifida. Neurosurg Clin N Am. 1995;6(2):203–18.
26. Apkon SD, Grady R, Hart S, et al. Advances in the care of children with spina bifida. Adv Pediatr Infect Dis. 2014;61(1):33–74.
27. North T, Cheong A, Steinbok P, Radic JA. Trends in incidence and long-term outcomes of myelomeningocele in British Columbia. Childs Nerv Syst. 2018;34(4):717–24.
28. Phillips LA, Burton JM, Evans SH. Spina bifida management. Curr Probl Pediatr Adolesc Health Care. 2017;47(7):173–7.
29. McLone DG. Technique for closure of myelomeningocele. Childs Brain. 1980;6(2):65–73.
30. Begeerl JH, Meihuizen de Regt MJ, HogenEsch I, Ter Weeme CA, Mooij JJ, Vencken LM. Progressive neurological deficit in children with spina bifida aperta. Z Kinderchir. 1986;41(suppl 1):13–5.
31. Moldenhauer JS, Adzick NS. Fetal surgery for myelomeningocele: after the Management of Myelomeningocele Study (MOMS). Semin Fetal Neonatal Med. 2017;22(6):360–6.
32. Adzick NS, Thom EA, Spong CY, et al. A randomized trial of prenatal versus postnatal repair of myelomeningocele. N Engl J Med. 2011;364(11):993–1004.
33. Brock JW 3rd, Carr MC, Adzick NS, et al. Bladder function after fetal surgery for myelomeningocele. Pediatrics. 2015;136(4):e906–13.
34. Farmer DL, Thom EA, Brock JW 3rd, et al. The management of myelomeningocele study: full cohort 30-month pediatric outcomes. Am J Obstet Gynecol. 2018;218(2):256.e1–256.e13.
35. Chan YY, Sandlin SK, Kurzrock EA. Urological outcomes of myelomeningocele and lipomeningocele. Curr Urol Rep. 2017;18(5):35.
36. Bowman RM, McLone DG, Grant JA, Tomita T, Ito JA. Spina bifida outcome: a 25-year prospective. Pediatr Neurosurg. 2001;34(3):114–20.
37. DG ML. Continuing concepts in the management of spina bifida. Pediatr Neurosurg. 1992;18(5–6):254–6.
38. French BN. The embryology of spinal dysraphism. Clin Neurosurg. 1983;30:295–340.
39. Bao N, Chen ZH, Gu S, Chen QM, Jin HM, Shi CR. Tight filum terminale syndrome in children: analysis based on positioning of the conus and absence or presence of lumbosacral lipoma. Childs Nerv Syst. 2007;23(10):1129–34.
40. McLendon RE, Oakes WJ, Heinz ER, Yeates AE, Burger PC. Adipose tissue in the filum terminale: a computed tomographic finding that may indicate tethering of the spinal cord. Neurosurgery. 1988;22(5):873–6.
41. Yamada S, Sanders DC, Maeda G. Oxidative metabolism during and following ischemia of cat spinal cord. Neurol Res. 1981;3(1):1–16.
42. Yamada S, Knerium DS, Mandybur GM, Schultz RL, Yamada BS. Pathophysiology of tethered cord syndrome and other complex factors. Neurol Res. 2004;26(7):722–6.
43. Oakes WJ. The borderlands of the primary tethered cord syndrome. Clin Neurosurg. 1996;43:188–202.
44. Rauzzino MJ, Iskandar BJ, Oakes WJ. Occult spinal dysraphism. Contemp Neurosurg. 1998;20:1–6.

45. Lapsiwala SB, Iskandar BJ. The tethered cord syndrome in adults with spina bifida occulta. Neurol Res. 2004;26(7):735–40.
46. Kulkarni AV, Pierre-Kahn A, Zerah M. Conservative management of asymptomatic spinal lipomas of the conus. Neurosurgery. 2004;54(4):868–73. discussion 873–875
47. Hoffman H, Taecholarn C, Hendrick E, et al. Lipomyelomeningoceles and their treatment. Concepts Pediatr Neurosurg. 1985;5:107–17.
48. Ammerman BJ, Henry JM, De Girolami U, Earle KM. Intradural lipomas of the spinal cord. A clinicopathological correlation. J Neurosurg. 1976;44(3):331–6.
49. French BN. Abnormal development of the central nervous system. In: McLauren RL, Schut L, Venes JL, editors. Pediatric neurosurgery, vol. 9. 2nd ed. Philadelphia: WB Saunders; 1989.
50. McLone DG, Thompson DNP. Lipomas of the spine. In: Pediatric neurosurgery: surgery of the developing nervous system. Philadelphia: WB Saunders; 2001. p. 289–301.
51. Chapman PH. Congenital intraspinal lipomas: anatomic considerations and surgical treatment. Childs Brain. 1982;9(1):37–47.
52. Chapman PH, Davis KR. Surgical treatment of spinal lipomas in childhood. Pediatr Neurosurg. 1993;19(5):267–75.
53. Pang D, Zovickian J, Oviedo A. Long-term outcome of total and near-total resection of spinal cord lipomas and radical reconstruction of the neural placode: part I—surgical technique. Neurosurgery. 2009;65(3):511–28. discussion 528–529
54. Walsh JW, Osterdock RJ. Lipomyelomeningocele. In: Winn HR, editor. Youmans neurological surgery. 5th ed. Philadelphia: Elsevier; 2004. p. 3229–44.
55. McLone DG, Mutluer S, Naidich TP. Lipomeningoceles of the conus medullaris. Concepts Pediatr Neurosurg. 1983;3:170–7.
56. Hoffman HJ, Taecholarn C, Hendrick EB, Humphreys RP. Management of lipomyelomeningoceles. Experience at the Hospital for Sick children, Toronto. J Neurosurg. 1985;62(1):1–8.
57. Villarejo FJ, Blasquez MG, Guierrez-Diaz JA. Intraspinal lipomas in children. Childs Brain. 1976;2(6):361–70.
58. Sutton LN. Lipomyelomeningocele. Neurosurg Clin N Am. 1995;6(2):325–38.
59. Bruce DA, Schut L. Spinal lipomas in infancy and childhood. Childs Brain. 1979;5(3):192–203.
60. James CCM, Lassman LP. Spina bifida occulta: orthopedic, radiological and neurosurgical aspects. London: Academic; 1981.
61. Kanev PM, Bierbrauer KS. Reflections on the natural history of lipomyelomeningocele. Pediatr Neurosurg:–140.
62. Schut L, Bruce DA, Sutton LN. The management of the child with a lipomyelomeningocele. Clin Neurosurg. 1983;30:464–76.
63. Pierre-Kahn A, Lacombe J, Pichon J, et al. Intraspinal lipomas with spina bifida. Prognosis and treatment in 73 cases. J Neurosurg. 1986;65(6):756–61.
64. McLone DG, Naidich TP. Laser resection of fifty spinal lipomas. Neurosurgery. 1986;18(5):611–5.
65. Finn MA, Walker ML. Spinal lipomas: clinical spectrum, embryology, and treatment. Neurosurg Focus. 2007;23(2):E10–2.
66. Atala A, Bauer SB, Dyro FM, et al. Bladder functional changes resulting from lipomyelomeningocele repair. J Urol. 1992;148(2 Pt 2):592–4.
67. Pang D, Dias MS, Ahab-Barmada M. Split cord malformation: part I: a unified theory of embryogenesis for double spinal cord malformations. Neurosurgery. 1992;31(3):451–80.
68. Garzo-Mercado R. Diastematomyelia and intramedullary epidermoid spinal tumor combined with extra-dural teratoma in an adult. J Neurosurg. 1983;58(6):954–8.
69. Mahapatra AK, Gupta DK. Split cord malformations: a clinical study of 254 patients and a proposal for a new clinical-imaging classification. J Neurosurg. 2005;103(suppl 6):531–6.
70. Pang D, Wilberger JF Jr. Tethered cord syndrome in adults. J Neurosurg. 1982;57(1):32–47.
71. Pang D. Split cord malformation: part II: clinical syndrome. Neurosurgery. 1992;31(3):481–500.
72. Ein SH, Mancer K, Adeyemi SD. Malignant sacrococcygeal teratoma—endodermal sinus, yolk sac tumor—in infants and children: a 32-year review. J Pediatr Surg. 1985;20(5):473–7.

73. Gumerlock MK, Spollen LE, Nelson MJ, Bishop RC, Cooperstock MS. Cervical neurenteric fistula causing recurrent meningitis in Klippel-Feil sequence: case report and literature review. Pediatr Infect Dis J. 1991;10(7):532–5.
74. Garg N, Sampath S, Yasha TC, Chandramouli BA, Devi I, Kovoor JME. Is total excision of spinal neurenteric cysts possible? Br J Neurosurg. 2008;22(2):241–51.
75. Riviérez M, Buisson G, Kujas M, et al. Intramedullary neurenteric cyst without any associated malformation. One case evaluated by RMI and electron microscopic study. Acta Neurochir. 1997;139(9):887–90.
76. Kole MJ, Fridley JS, Jea A, Bollo RJ. Currarino syndrome and spinal dysraphism. J Neurosurg Pediatr. 2014;13(6):685–9.
77. Beyazal M. An asymptomatic large anterior sacral meningocele in a patient with a history of gestation: a case report with radiological findings. Case Rep Radiol. 2013;2013:842620.

Chapter 19
Persistent Terminal Ventricle

Yasmin Ahmadi, Tabarak Qassim, Ahmed Kazerooni, Farhan Rana, Usama AlDallal, Leen Rikan Azzam, Maryam Salman, K. G. Akashnath, and Narjiss Aji

Test your learning and check your understanding of this book's contents: use the "Springer Nature Flashcards" app to access questions using ▶ https://sn.pub/QCsfpd.
To use the app, please follow the instructions in Chap. 1.

19.1 Introduction

The ventriculus terminalis also known as terminal ventricle of Krause or the fifth ventricle is defined as an expansion of the conus' central canal, bordered by ependymal cells containing CSF. It is considered a normal pattern related to the embryological development of the neural tube between the seventh and the eighth week and it is supposed to regress during the following differentiation period [1, 2]. In rare cases, an unsuccessful regression can happen and may be visualized by radiological investigations finding in children. This condition, which etiopathogenesis is still

Y. Ahmadi · T. Qassim (✉) · F. Rana · U. AlDallal · L. R. Azzam · M. Salman
K. G. Akashnath
School of Medicine, Royal College of Surgeons in Ireland-Bahrain, Busaiteen, Bahrain
e-mail: 18203205@rcsi.com; 17221587@rcsi.com; 17211638@rcsi.com

A. Kazerooni
College of Medicine and Medical Sciences, Arabian Gulf University, Manama, Bahrain

N. Aji
Faculty of Medicine and Pharmacy of Rabat, Rabat, Morocco

K. F. AlAli, H. T. Hashim (eds.), *Congenital Spine Malformations*,
https://doi.org/10.1007/978-3-031-59031-3_19

debatable, can be responsible for wide neurological symptoms ranging from sciatica to gait disturbance. Literature suggests that management can conservative or surgical depending if the patient is symptomatic or not [3].

19.2 Pathogenesis and Pathophysiology

The terminal ventricle is a space lined by ependymal cells which is formed as a part of normal embryogenesis of the neuronal tube within day 43–48 of development. It is thought to be shaped by the canalization of the conus medullaris, located in the caudal end of the spinal cord. Followed by successive regression of that cavity during the differentiation phase. During the latter phase the caudal neural tube and the notochord fuse to form the caudal cell mass. Next, vacuoles start to form within this mass which results in the development of a cavity called "The Terminal Ventricle". On some occasions, this cavity can persist until adulthood. This persistent terminal ventricle usually contains cerebrospinal fluid and was used to be thought to have direct connection with the central canal of the anterior portion of the spinal canal [4–11]. However, the latter statement has been refuted by ECG-gated SPAMM-MR imaging studies which are used to indicate cerebrospinal fluid motion within the spinal cord. Sigal et al. reported absence of pulsatile motion within the persistent terminal ventricle indicating its lack of connection with the central canal [7, 12].

19.3 Clinical Presentation

Patients with persistent terminal ventricle or ventriculus terminalis (VT) typically present with a wide range of symptoms and they can be categorized into three groups (Table 19.1) depending on the neurological manifestation involved [13]. Type I presents as nonspecific complaints or neurological manifestations such as sciatica, lower back pain, and lower limb pain [13]. Type 1 can be further classified into type Ia indicating a nonprogressive nature in the neurological presentation and type Ib indicating a progressive and worsening nature of the neurological deficit [13]. Type II VT presents with focal neurological deficits including sensory deficits, altered deep tendon reflexes (areflexia, hyporeflexia, brisk reflex, or hyperreflexia),

Table 19.1 The classification of the symptoms grading

Type I	Type II	Type III
Lower back pain	Gait disturbance	Sphincter dysfunction (bowel or bladder)
Sciatica	Paresis	
Inferior limb pain	Sensory disturbance	
	Altered reflexes	
	Muscular atrophy	

Table 19.2 The neurological classification of the malformation

Sensory deficits	Motor deficits
Unilateral or bilateral lower limb pain	Gait disturbance
Sciatica	Muscular atrophy
Lower back pain	Paresis
Paraesthesia	Anal and bladder sphincter dysfunction
	Altered reflexes

gait disturbances, muscular atrophy, and paresis [13]. Type III presents with signs of urorectal sphincter dysfunction such as bowel and/or bladder incontinence [13] (Table 19.2).

19.4 Differential Diagnosis and Diagnosis

In the distal central spinal cord canal, VT is shown as a cystic lesion without aberrant cord signaling [14]. It is usually an asymptomatic and incidental finding in adults. The discovery and diagnosis of ventriculus terminalis can be greatly aided by dorsolumbar magnetic resonance imaging (dorsolumbar MRI). It effectively distinguishes the condition from other lesions affecting the cord or conus with signal intensity characteristics that match CSF on all sequences, showing the conus medullaris as a homogenous non-enhancing cystic dilatation [7, 15].

If the cystic lesion of the conus medullaris contains septation and edema, a crucial differential diagnosis of spinal neoplasm should be taken into account [12]. A filar cyst, a smooth, dilated chamber within the conus medullaris that is discovered by coincidence during fetal lumbar sonography in the filum terminale, is a top differential diagnosis to be considered [16].

Syringohydromyelia, cystic intramedullary tumors [14], syringomyelia [17], artefact (which may be caused by pulsation from cord motion or truncation at dark/bright signal interfaces) [4], and cystic neoplasm [15] are among the other potential diagnoses. Furthermore, ependymoma, astrocytoma, hemangioblastoma and oligodendroglioma have all been differential diagnoses linked to VT [15]. A possibility of an epidermoid congenital lesion can be considered if there is history of spina bifida with spinal cord tethering or if there is a dermal sinus tract present in children [14].

19.5 Investigations

19.5.1 Imaging

A persistent terminal ventricle can be identified as a cystic mass present between the point of the conus terminalis until the filum terminale. MRI is the diagnostic imaging form of choice through which persistent terminal ventricle is identified.

In newborns, this cystic structure has an approximate diameter of 8–10 mm longitudinally and 2–4 mm transversely [7]. Later in childhood, this cystic structure tends to continue remaining visible.

In children under the age of 5, MRI depicts an ovoid, non-intense dilatation of the central canal inside the conus terminalis. This dilatation is said to be a normal developmental phenomenon [14].

In adults, unusual features are observed on MRI. The size of the cysts is between 15 and 68 mm, with a mean of 32.67 ± 18.5 mm. The lesions are located within the central spinal cord, in the lower thoracic end at T11/T12 [12].

MRI imaging typically shows the following fluid signal characteristics [18]:

T1—Hypointensity seen
T2—Hyperintensity seen

19.5.2 Sonography

Five neonates with ventriculus terminalis who were scanned and followed up after 3 months depicted normal-appearing conus medullaris terminating in the normal position of L1–L2, with ambulant nerve roots. Apparent division of the central echo complex was seen within the Conus terminalis; an unusual appearance [19].

Sonography repeated at 3 months depicted no interval change of the hypoechogenic or divided central echo complex in two of the infants [19].

19.6 Management

The management of persistent terminal ventricle is still a controversial topic, due to its rarity. However, various studies have used similar methods in managing this disease, which consists of merely treating patients who are symptomatic with neurological deficits or a deteriorating state. Asymptomatic patients do not usually require treatment. The mainstay treatment of symptomatic patients is surgery [3].

A management flow-chart was proposed by De Moura Batista et al. and adjusted by Kawanishi et al., which states that asymptomatic patients should be managed conservatively, and that surgery should be reserved for symptomatic patients. Additionally, if the patient presents with an increased dimension of the cyst or worsening neurological condition, they then would be counseled to undergo the surgery. Nonetheless, the surgical management for symptomatic patients are deemed to be an effective option for the relief of their symptoms and not as a curative option. The chart states that there are four types of patients, which consist of [1]:

Type 1a—stable patients that present with non-specific symptoms
Type 1b—patients presenting with non-specific worsening symptoms
Type 2—patients presenting with focal neurological deficits
Type 3—patients presenting with sphincter dysfunctions

Initially, those patients first undertake preliminary assessments before management is conducted, which consists of an MRI of the whole spine and the brain to rule-out other pathologies (e.g. brain/spinal tumor; chiari malformation). After the preoperative imaging is conducted and verified of ventriculus terminalis diagnosis, Type 1a patients start their conservative management, then are followed up after 3 months. The follow-up consists of an additional clinical examination and MRI of the spine and brain [20].

A large cohort study completed on patients with ventriculus terminalis concluded that surgical treatment should be reserved for type 1b, II, and III patients to partially or completely relieve their symptoms. Some research also suggested that patients with type 1a lesions should be offered surgery as a primary prevention method to decrease the risk of cyst growth and associated neurological deterioration. In this case, if type 1a patients reject the surgical route, they should be closely monitored as cyst growth and symptom progression may occur rapidly [21].

The commonly conducted procedure is a combined cyst fenestration through laminectomy and a small midline myeletomy; after the drainage of the cavity, the cyst is marsupialized to obtain a good CSF flow. Cyst fenestration has been shown to result in complete clinical recovery in 52% of cases and partial recovery in 43% of cases [22].

Furthermore, placement of a cyst-subarachnoid shunt can also be conducted. The shunt's aim is to exclude any concerns of closure of the cyst wall and reduces the risk of postoperative cyst recurrence. In the cohort study, patients who did not undergo the shunt, later presented with partial cyst recurrence, which led to another surgical fenestration to be conducted due to the symptom recurrence. Although, this method is shown to be an effective and safe management option, there are alternatives with better advantages and shorter hospital stay and are non-invasive with no postoperative surgical site symptoms, such as percutaneous aspiration of CSF during real-time MRI, but only limited evidence is available to confirm its effectiveness. However, this alternative method may be hazardous due to a higher risk of damaging the rich perimedullary vascular network [21].

19.7 Conclusion

Formation of the terminal ventricle is a natural process occurring during embryogenesis of the neuronal tube between days 43 and 48. At a later stage, a cavity begins to form in it and it is when it persists and doesn't regress that it becomes pathogenic.

The clinical presentation varies from nonspecific symptoms to focal neurological deficits or urorectal sphincter dysfunction. When investigating VT in newborns, MRI is the investigation of choice which would display the cystic structure with a longitudinal diameter of 8–10 mm and a transverse diameter of 2–4 mm. In children below the age of 5, an ovoid, non-enhancing, smooth dilatation of the central canal within the conus medullaris would be seen. In adults, unusual features are observed on the MRI. The lesions would be located within the central spinal cord, in the lower thoracic end at T11/T12, varying in size between 15 and 68 mm. Management of VT depends on the patient's clinical presentation. While the asymptomatic ones do not require treatment, the symptomatic patients displaying neurological deficits or a deteriorating state undergo surgery. Management of those patients initially starts with an MRI of the entire spine and brain to rule out other pathologies. Afterwards, the patients would be divided into four classifications depending on their presentations and state as shown in the chart. Prognosis of this illness is insufficiently documented in literature.

Multiple Choice Questions

1. During which days of embryogenesis does the terminal ventricle start to form?
2. Which part of the spinal cord usually contains the terminal ventricle?
3. What are the two phases that form the terminal ventricle?
4. What type of cells line the terminal ventricle?
5. During the differentiation phase, the caudal neural tube and notochord fuse to form the?
6. What forms inside this caudal cell mass?
7. The persistent terminal ventricle usually contains inside of it?
8. If the cystic lesion of the conus medullaris contains septation and edema, what is your primary differential?
9. What's the primary investigation done before initiating management?
10. For the patients that require surgical treatment, what is the surgical procedure conducted for them?
11. In management, surgery is reserved for which types of patients?
12. What are the four classifications that determine the management?

Answers

1. *Days 43–48*
2. *Conus medullaris*
3. *Canalization and regression*
4. *Ependymal cells*
5. *Caudal cell mass*
6. *Vacuoles*
7. *Cerebrospinal fluid*
8. *Spinal neoplasm*
9. *MRI of the whole spine and the brain*
10. *Combined cyst fenestration through laminectomy and a small midline myeletomy*
11. *Types 1b, 2 and 3*
12. *The classification is:*

    (a) *Type 1a—stable patients that present with non-specific symptoms*
    (b) *Type 1b—patients presenting with non-specific worsening symptoms*
    (c) *Type 2—patients presenting with focal neurological deficits*
    (d) *Type 3—patients presenting with sphincter dysfunctions*

References

1. Nunes RH, Abello AL, Castillo M. Critical findings in neuroradiology. Springer International Publishing; 2016.
2. Albright AL, Pollack IF, Adelson PD. Principles and practice of pediatric neurosurgery. Thieme Publishing Group; 2007.
3. Fletcher-Sandersjöö A, Edström E, Bartek J Jr, Elmi-Terander A. Surgical treatment for symptomatic ventriculus terminalis: case series and a literature review. Acta Neurochir (Wien). 2019;161(9):1901–8.
4. Kernohan JW. The ventriculus terminalis: its growth and development. J Comp Neurol. 1924;38(1):107–25.
5. Van Rillaer O, Vandaele P, Ramboer K. Malformative persistence of terminal ventricle. JBR-BTR. 2009;92(3):178–9.
6. Celli P, D'Andrea G, Trillò G, Roperto R, Acqui M, Ferrante L. Cyst of the medullary conus: malformative persistence of terminal ventricle or compressive dilatation? Neurosurg Rev. 2002;25(1–2):103–6.
7. Sigal R, Denys A, Halimi P, Shapeero L, Doyon D, Boudghène F. Ventriculus terminalis of the conus medullaris: MR imaging in four patients with congenital dilatation. Am J Neuroradiol. 1991;12(4):733–7.
8. Dhillon RS, McKelvie PA, Wang YY, Han T, Murphy M. Cystic lesion of the ventriculus terminalis in an adult. J Clin Neurosci. 2010;17(12):1601–3.
9. Agrillo U, Tirendi MN, Nardi PV. Symptomatic cystic dilatation of V ventricle: case report and review of the literature. Eur Spine J. 1997;6(4):281–3.
10. Matsubayashi R, Uchino A, Kato A, Kudo S, Sakai S, Murata S. Cystic dilatation of ventriculus terminalis in adults: MRI. Neuroradiology. 1998;40(1):45–7.
11. Nassar SI, Correll JW, Housepian EM. Intramedullary cystic lesions of the conus medullaris. J Neurol Neurosurg Psychiatry. 1968;31(2):106–9.
12. Suh SH, Chung TS, Lee SK, Cho YE, Kim KS. Ventriculus terminalis in adults: unusual magnetic resonance imaging features and review of the literature. Korean J Radiol. 2012;13(5):557–63.
13. Ganau M, Talacchi A, Cecchi PC, Ghimenton C, Gerosa M, Faccioli F. Cystic dilation of the ventriculus terminalis: clinical article. J Neurosurg Spine. 2012;17(1):86–92.
14. Coleman LT, Zimmerman RA, Rorke LB. Ventriculus terminalis of the conus medullaris: MR findings in children. AJNR Am J Neuroradiol. 1995;16(7):1421–6.
15. Dullerud R, Server A, Berg-Johnsen J. MR imaging of ventriculus terminalis of the conus medullaris. A report of two operated patients and a review of the literature. Acta Radiol. 2003;44(4):444–6.
16. Irani N, Goud AR, Lowe LH. Isolated filar cyst on lumbar spine sonography in infants: a case-control study. Pediatr Radiol. 2006;36(12):1283–8.
17. Ciappetta P, D'Urso PI, Luzzi S, Ingravallo G, Cimmino A, Resta L. Cystic dilation of the ventriculus terminalis in adults. J Neurosurg Spine. 2008;8(1):92–9.
18. Radswiki T, Al Kabbani A, Botz B, et al. Ventriculus terminalis. Reference article. Radiopaedia.org. https://doi.org/10.53347/rID-12435. Accessed on 16 Dec 2022.
19. Kriss VM, Kriss TC, Babcock DS. The ventriculus terminalis of the spinal cord in the neonate: a normal variant on sonography. AJR Am J Roentgenol. 1995;165(6):1491–3.
20. Severino R, Severino P. Surgery or not? A case of ventriculus terminalis in an adult patient. J Spine Surg. 2017;3(3):475–80.
21. Mateusz Szostak MW, Śniegocki M, Siedlecki Z, Nowak K, Grzyb S, Gromadzki B, Grzonkowska M. Ventriculus terminalis cyst—case report and literature review. Eur J Mol Clin Med. 2020;7(10):1027–31.
22. Woodley-Cook J, Konieczny M, Spears J. The slowly enlarging ventriculus terminalis. Pol J Radiol. 2016;81:529–31.

Chapter 20
Terminal Myelocystocele

Mahdi Abdalhusain and Abdullah Alsayedomar

Test your learning and check your understanding of this book's contents: use the "Springer Nature Flashcards" app to access questions using ▶ https://sn.pub/QCsfpd.

To use the app, please follow the instructions in Chap. 1.

20.1 Introduction

Terminal myelocystocele (TMC) is a rare congenital spinal dysraphism characterized by a herniation through a posterior spina bifida that consists of a cystic dilatation of the spinal cord's central canal. These lesions develop from abnormalities of the caudal cell mass. They are characterized by a massive, well-covered lumbosacral mass comprising fat, cerebrospinal fluid (CSF), and neural tissue. The central canal opens into a hollow lined with ependymal cells and is filled with CSF, while the spinal cord herniates through the dysraphic spine and ends at a neural placode. The lump may occasionally grow to enormous proportions, leaving the patient with aesthetic deformities in addition to neurological consequences from the cord's tethering. Anomalies of the anorectal system, lower genitourinary system, and vertebrae can also be present in TMC. Anal atresia, cloacal exstrophy, lordosis, scoliosis, and incomplete sacral agenesis are associated malformations [1]. It accounts for 5% of closed spinal dysraphism in those who have a noticeable back mass [2]. Congenital

M. Abdalhusain (✉) · A. Alsayedomar
University of Malta, Msida, Malta
e-mail: mahdi.abdalhusain.17@um.edu.mt; abdullah.a.alsayed-omar.16@um.edu.mt

K. F. AlAli, H. T. Hashim (eds.), *Congenital Spine Malformations*,
https://doi.org/10.1007/978-3-031-59031-3_20

abnormalities occur as a result of an error occurring throughout the complex process of development. As a result, these anomalies typically display a wide range of morphology. Finding two distinct cases with comparable morphologies or the same case with radically different looks is not unusual. Therefore, grouping congenital abnormalities based on gross morphology might be unclear. The issue surrounding the categorization of TMC, which displays many diverse morphologies, was resolved by studying its embryogenesis [3].

20.2 Etiology and Pathogenesis

TMC is believed to emerge randomly instead of being familial in nature. However, teratogens such as hydantoin, loperamide hydrochloride, and retinoic acid have been implicated as the cause of this condition. No sex predominance was noted in patients with TMC.

The spinal cord normally develops in two phases. The more distal cord conus medullaris and filum terminale develop via canalization and retrogressive differentiation, whereas the segment from the medulla to mid lumbar region develops through neurulation. Numerous locations start the neurulation process, which moves both directions. At around 24 and 27 days, respectively, the anterior and posterior neuropores close. The neural tube's elongation caudal to the posterior neuropore is known as canalization. The notochord and neural epithelium join together to produce the caudal mass. Within this mass, microcysts start to form at around 30 days and eventually unite to create an ependyma-lined tube that joins the neural tube. The caudal neural tube diminishes in size around day 38 as a result of cell necrosis. The distal conus medullaris, filum terminale, and ventriculus terminalis are formed by this retrogressive differentiation. It is believed that TMCs form due to spontaneous closure of the caudal end of the neural tube. CSF causes the caudal end of the neural tube to enlarge, which dilates the ventriculus terminalis and causes the dorsal mesenchyme to rupture. Dilatation of the ventriculus terminalis and inability of the posterior elements to grow causes the formation of the meningocele [4]. TMCs may develop at any level of the spine. Depending on their location and post-operative pathological findings, they are divided into terminal and non-terminal lesions [5].

20.3 Diagnosis

20.3.1 History and Clinical Presentation

Compared to newborns with meningomyelocele, neonates with TMC exhibit less clinically significant symptoms [6]. The diagnosis is determined quickly after delivery because the bulge on the sacral region is not minor. Numerous individuals present with symptoms during their physical examinations and during extensive urological or electrophysiological studies at the time of diagnosis, although neurologically normal patients are also seen. Most patients that were diagnosed with TMC later in life had symptoms such as neurogenic bladder and lower extremity motor deficits. Therefore, it is advised that surgical treatment be taken into account even for individuals who are asymptomatic. Other possible symptoms include sensory loss and bowel incontinence. Enlargement of the cyst is a distinctive clinical characteristic that should be taken into account in the therapy of TMC since it serves as a warning indicator for the quick progression of neurological impairments. A foot deformity that develops in less than two months is an example of how quickly the progression may occur. The spinal cord may be directly stretched by the cyst's growth, which would quickly deteriorate the condition [3]. Despite the fact that just a few studies have linked TMC to hindbrain abnormalities (i.e., Chiari malformations), the majority of studies have shown no connection between the two. TMC appears to be sporadic in that there is no proof that it is a hereditary disorder [6, 7].

20.3.2 Physical Examination

Findings of physical examinations of patients with TMC often show variable deficits. Most common finding is a lumbosacral mass that is covered with irregular skin [8]. Other possible findings include muscle weakness due to wasting and shortening of a single leg, smaller buttocks on one side, a shorter or a more highly arched foot. Some patients exhibit either brisk or absent knee and ankle reflexes and plantar response on one side. Others exhibit sensory loss over a particular dermatome such as S2. Scoliosis is another condition that can be seen in patients with TMC [2].

20.3.3 Neuroimaging

MRI of the lumbosacral spinal cord exhibit a number of essential characteristics that are consistent and seen in most patients with TMCs, as well as other results that are optional and not characteristic of this condition. The primary defining characteristic of TMC is an enlarged spinal cord that protrudes dorsally from the spinal canal and grows into the TMC. The flared portion of the trumpet resembles a three-dimensional cone, with the broad base adhering to the subcutaneous fat layer of the overlying skin and the tip toward the side of the spinal canal. The fluid-filled chamber is most often separated from the surrounding fat by a thin but noticeable layer of tissue that is continuous with the trumpet's inner lining. A continuation of the extraspinal cystic cavity with varying degrees of hydromyelia in the intraspinal part of the caudal spinal cord is one of the optional characteristics of TMC [7]. The hydromyelia's width and length can also range from average to exceptionally high [3]. High dimensions of the subarachnoid CSF space around the extruded neck of the terminating spinal cord are another optional characteristic of TMC. In some circumstances, the intraspinal portion of this space could reach exceptional sizes [7].

20.3.4 Other Investigations

Renal scans, ultrasounds, and tests of renal function are used to assess urinary tract function [9]. The lumbosacral mass can be investigated using an ultrasound scan in order to view the cystic swelling and the meninges. A fetus with a cystic growth over the lower back should be evaluated for TMC, especially if there is a "cyst within a cyst" appearance on ultrasound. It is necessary to take into account other cystic masses in the lumbosacral region such as myelomeningoceles, meningoceles and cystic sacrococcygeal teratoma. Examining the cyst walls, intracystic contents, fetal head, and the presence or absence of spinal dysraphism can help differentiate between myelomeningocele, meningocele, cystic sacrococcygeal teratoma, and TMC if a cystic mass is discovered along the lumbosacral area on an antenatal ultrasound [10].

20.4 Management

It is stated that surgical repair of the myelocystocele is the treatment for TMC [11]. Improved outcomes result from immediate surgical repair [9]. Under this heading, we will cover surgical procedure steps and pre- and post-operative observation in selected patients.

20.4.1 Surgical Procedure

The surgical team should arrange the patient in a face-down (prone) position. A midline vertical or lateral semicircular skin incision is possible around the lumbar mass [11]. When the dura is accessible, a durotomy should be performed to expose the neck of the herniated mass and the cord cephalic and caudal to the neck. Following this, the mass is divided to expose the neural placode, which is subsequently dissected at its periphery and rebuilt. In the meanwhile, the surgeon would use electrophysiological studies to identify the conducting rootlets by stimulating the spinal cord. Following this, the mass is dissected, the inside is exposed, and it is stimulated to detect the dysfunctional fibers, so providing a good outline of the area to be mutilated. Finally, the dura must be repaired with bovine pericardium to enhance the ratio of cord to sac [3].

20.4.2 Pre- and Post-operative Observations

Tandon et al. and Gupta et al., described their patient's outcomes before and after surgical intervention. Tandon et al. recorded 30 male and female patients ranging in age from 1 month to 15 years within 10 years between 2000 and 2010. Males made up around 53% of the cohort, which consists of 16 individuals. Only two-thirds exhibited symptoms. All of them displayed lumbosacral enlargement, although the percentages of the other symptoms varied. After resection of the myelocystocele, symptoms improved in 90% of patients (27), while two patients with total flaccid paraplegia exhibited no change and one patient experienced a worsening of symptoms. Almost half of the patients suffered problems, including pseudomeningococcal, cerebrospinal fluid (CSF) leak, pyrexia of unexplained origin, meningitis, and surgical site infection [1].

Between 1998 and 2004, Gupta et al. reported 17 multisex patients diagnosed with TMC. The group consisted primarily of women (about 11 patients). The average age of the patients is about 1 year and 8 months (between 2 and 5 years). Similarly, all registered cases revealed lumbosacral cysts of varying mean sizes covered by normal skin. There were no concomitant symptoms in 9 patients (52.9%), while the remainder presented with symptoms including lower limb involvement, flaccid paraplegia, and autonomic dysfunction (constipation and urinary incontinence). Of the latter, 3 had both UI and constipation, whereas the remaining 5 had only UI. After removal of the mass and detethering of the spinal cord, the nine patients who had only Lumbosacral mass remained normal. However, six individuals in the other group demonstrated improvement, while only three continued to exhibit symptoms, two of which deteriorated and one remained unaltered. The former two developed cerebrospinal fluid (CSF) leakage, and one of those patients developed meningitis [12].

20.4.3 Prevention

In general, malformations of the central nervous system can be averted using simple but limited measures. According to Ansari et al., women of reproductive age should take folic acid. In addition, they underlined the importance of prenatal screening programs [13].

20.5 Complications and Prognosis

Prior to the 1980s, it was advised that individuals with TMC should not be treated, leaving the patients to die. Nowadays, with the advent of new surgical methods, however, life expectancy has increased and the quality of life has improved. The most often reported consequences are lumbar mass, autonomic dysfunction and motor weakness [14]. According to Pang et al., spinal cord tethering would result in rapid growth of the bulk followed by health decline. This is a surgical emergency that requires immediate surgical intervention [7]. Additionally, the data suggests an increase in the average period of hospitalization, which now averages 64 days [14]. This would also raise the incidence of hospital-acquired illnesses among these individuals [15].

Multiple Choice Questions

1. **The neurenteric canal forms in the region of the**:

   A. Hypoblast
   B. Primitive pit
   C. Yolk sac
   D. Amniotic cavity

2. **Posterior enteric remnants include all of the following except**:

   A. Diverticulum
   B. Sinus
   C. Cyst
   D. Diastematomyelia

3. **The following statement concerns the posterior enteric fistula**:

   A. The embryonic fistula is fully intact
   B. The dorsal part of the embryonic fistula is intact
   C. The ventral part of the embryonic fistula is intact
   D. The intermediate part of the embryonic fistula is intact

4. **A neonate with a dorsal enteric fistula will present at birth with**:

   A. Meconium coming out of the bowel ostium cranially
   B. Meconium coming out of the bowel ostium at the back
   C. Meconium coming out of the bowel ostium at the front
   D. Meconium coming out of the bowel ostium caudally

5. **Histopathological examination of the posterior enteric remnant reveals that its walls contain**:

   A. Columnar epithelium
   B. Simple squamous epithelium
   C. Stratified squamous keratinized epithelium
   D. Pseudostratified Columnar epithelium

6. **Dorsal enteric fistulas are classified as**

   A. Cranial defects
   B. Open neural tube defects
   C. Closed neural tube defects
   D. Disorder of notochord formation

7. **The notochord formation begins when the cells in the primitive streak migrate**

   A. Cranially
   B. Caudally
   C. Laterally
   D. Transversely

8. **Split notochord syndrome represents an extremely rare and pleomorphic form of spinal dysraphism characterized by**

   A. A persistent communication between the endoderm and the mesoderm
   B. A persistent communication between the endoderm and the ectoderm
   C. A persistent communication between the ectoderm and mesoderm
   D. A persistent communication between the ectoderm, endoderm, and mesoderm

9. **Which neuroimaging technique can aid in the diagnosis of dorsal enteric fistula**?

   A. Ultrasound
   B. X-ray
   C. CT scan
   D. PET scan

10. **What is the most common location of the dorsal enteric fistula**?

   A. Colon
   B. Distal ileum
   C. Cecum
   D. Duodenum

Answers

1. B
2. D
3. A
4. B
5. A
6. C
7. A
8. B
9. C
10. A

References

1. Tandon V, Garg K, Mahapatra AK. Terminal myelocystocele: a series of 30 cases and review of the literature. Pediatr Neurosurg. 2012;48(4):229–35.
2. Cartmill M, Jaspan T, Punt J. Terminal myelocystocele: an unusual presentation. Pediatr Neurosurg. 2000;32(2):83–5.
3. Lee J, Kim K, Wang K. Terminal myelocystocele: pathoembryogenesis and clinical features. J Korean Neurosurg Soc. 2020;63(3):321–6.
4. Kumar R, Chandra A. Terminal myelocystocele. Indian J Pediatr. 2002;69(12):1083–6.
5. Muthukumar N. Terminal and nonterminal myelocystoceles. J Neurosurg Pediatr. 2007;107(2):87–97.
6. Meyer S, Morris G, Pretorius D, James H. Terminal myelocystocele: important differential diagnosis in the prenatal assessment of spina bifida. J Ultrasound Med. 1998;17(3):193–7.
7. Pang D, Zovickian J, Lee J, Moes G, Wang K. Terminal myelocystocele: surgical observations and theory of embryogenesis. Neurosurgery. 2012;70(6):1383–405.
8. Bansal S, Mahapatra A. "Giant" terminal myelocystocele: a rare variant of spinal dysraphism. Asian J Neurosurg. 2015;10(4):350–2.
9. Mirza B, Mahmood N, Ijaz L, Khawaja T, Aslam I, Sheikh A. Isolated terminal myelocystocele: a rare spinal dysraphism. APSP J Case Rep. 2022 [cited 15 September 2022]. Available from: https://pubmed.ncbi.nlm.nih.gov/22953270/.
10. AlSaffar H, Al Shammasi M, Ebrahim L. Antenatal ultrasound finding of a cystic Back mass in a fetus with terminal myelocystocele. Bahrain Med Bull. 2013 [cited 15 September 2022]. Available from: https://www.bahrainmedicalbulletin.com/june_2013/Antenatal_Ultrasound.pdf.
11. Massa D, Montivero N, Medina S. Terminal myelocystocele: surgical management. Surg Neurol Int. 2022;13:234.
12. Gupta D, Mahapatra A. Terminal myelocystoceles: a series of 17 cases. J Neurosurg Pediatr. 2005;103(4):344–52.
13. Ansari T, Ali L, Aziz T, Ara J, Liaquat N, Tahir H. Nutritional iron deficiency in women of child bearing age—what to do? J Ayub Med Coll Abbottabad. 2009;21(3):17–20 [cited 15 September 2022]. Available from: https://pubmed.ncbi.nlm.nih.gov/20929004/.
14. Choi S, McComb J. Long-term outcome of terminal myelocystocele patients. Pediatr Neurosurg. 2000;32(2):86–91.
15. Monegro AF, Muppidi V, Regunath H. Hospital acquired infections. StatPearls Publishing; 2019. Available from: https://www.ncbi.nlm.nih.gov/books/NBK441857/.

Chapter 21
Cervical Myelocystocele

Naseem Wajdi, Umniah Khajori, and Ali Tarik Abdul Wahid

Test your learning and check your understanding of this book's contents: use the "Springer Nature Flashcards" app to access questions using ▶ https://sn.pub/QCsfpd.
To use the app, please follow the instructions in Chap. 1.

21.1 Introduction

Cervical myelocystocele is a subtype of spinal dysraphism. It is a rare congenital malformation that constitutes about 1–5% of all neural tube defects [1] with around 15 cases reported in the literature [2].

Many researchers have tried to define cervical myelocystocele. As for Maclone et al., they defined it as a posterior midline mass, skin-covered, hence it is a type of 'closed' or 'occult' spinal dysraphism.

This lesion is also characterized by having a narrow spina bifida posteriorly with cysts that are filled with cerebrospinal fluid [3].

– Lesions with a stalk of glial or fibrovascular tissue in the cervical and upper thoracic region.

N. Wajdi (✉) · U. Khajori
College of Medicine, University of Baghdad, Baghdad, Iraq

A. T. A. Wahid
Neurosurgery, Department of Surgery, College of Medicine, University of Baghdad, Baghdad, Iraq
e-mail: alitarik@comed.uobaghdad.edu.iq

K. F. AlAli, H. T. Hashim (eds.), *Congenital Spine Malformations*,
https://doi.org/10.1007/978-3-031-59031-3_21

- Lesions comprising a meningocele with a herniated ependymal-lined cyst inside.
- Lesions without a stalk in the cervical and upper thoracic region (true meningoceles) [4].

Another classification proposed by Pang et al. splitting it into two categories:

- Lesions with fibroneurovascular stalk inside a rural sac but with limited posterior myeloschisis.
- Split spinal cord defects with two hemicords inside a dural sac [5].

Habibi et al. and Rossi et al. used another classification by dividing the lesions into two subgroups: fibroneurovascular stalks and myelocystoceles [6].

21.2 Presentations

Patients often present with a background of certain risk factors which may be genetic, environmental, or a combination of the two. One of the most prominent risk factors in literature is vitamin B12 (Folate) deficiency [7].

The presentation is usually at an early age after birth as a mass in the posterior neck region. Clinical examination of the patient may be normal except for the mass [8, 9]. The mass itself is usually tubular in shape protruding from the infant's neck and covered by thick skin and dystrophic squamous epithelium at the dome with margins of normal skin surrounding it [5, 10].

Symptoms and signs can range from pain, paranesthesia, upper motor weakness and bladder/bowel dysfunction [11].

Patients with cervical myelocystocele are neurologically preserved in comparison to those in the thoracolumbar or lumbosacral regions [12].

Certain conditions have been associated with cervical myelocystocele. For example, Chiari II malformations, hydrocephalus, aqueduct stenosis, neurenteric cyst, and lipoma of filum terminale [13].

21.3 Diagnosis

There's a vast array of differential diagnoses of neck masses in general. Often, we differentiate between them according to their site, size, consistency, and other mass features [14]. From the common reactive lymph nodes to the rare cervical spinal dysraphism in all of its forms.

In this case, magnetic resonance imaging (MRI) is the modality of choice in diagnosing such lesions, as it determines which subtype of cervical myelocystocele [15].

It also helps to identify any associated anomalies such as hydrocephalus, Klippel-Feil syndrome, craniovertebral junction anomalies, and Chiari malformations [16–18].

21.4 Treatment

Conservative management in such lesions risks progressive motor and sensory function compromise. Therefore, surgical exploration is the treatment option in such lesions, ideally within 3–6 months after birth to avoid neurological deterioration [19]. Patients experiencing sensory or motor symptoms, or having progressive neurological deficits, or having a rapidly increased size meningocele, should all undergo surgical management [20].

Surgical management aims at:

- Prevention of infection
- Cosmetical achievement
- Releasing the tethered cord, which is very important to reduce the symptoms and prevent the disease progression [6]

When approaching such cases, one should bear in mind whether the sac is ruptured or not, and whether primary hydrocephalus is present or not.

Non-terminal myelocystocele is the only type of closed spinal dysraphism that is associated with hydrocephalus [20].

Unruptured sacs can be operated on electively when the patient is medically and surgically fit for surgery even if it's delayed for a few months after birth. However, if any evidence of a ruptured sac, CSF leak, abnormal neurological exam, or failure to gain weight are observed, immediate surgical intervention is promoted, usually under general anesthesia, as these findings are considered an emergency [2].

If primary hydrocephalus is present, a ventriculoperitoneal (VP) shunt is indicated to relieve excess CSF fluid. If not, then the management is surgical according to patient's state as mentioned [21].

In a prone position, the lesion is marked and skin is opened via a simple vertical incision to gain access to the sac. Excess skin and sac tissue is then removed. A plain cervical X-ray should be taken preoperatively to minimize the skin incision. After dissecting the para-spinal muscles to view the spine, an intraoperative X-ray should be taken to confirm the cervical level. Then, the dural defect is repaired by primary closure and watertight closure technique. Afterwards, fibrin glue is used to strengthen the dural closure and minimize postoperative recurrence and CSF leak [20].

The simple excision of the meningocele sac through a linear incision and cutting the communication can provide a cosmetic repair. However, it will not prevent the neurological deterioration because of the tethering [22]. Failure to, or even partial detethering can result in bad prognosis with spastic and worsening limbs function [5].

Detethering of the cervical myelocystocele have shown symptomatic relief in affected patients and greater clinical outcomes [23].

Therefore, neurological deterioration prompts surgical re-exploration and resection of any remaining tethering.

21.5 Complications and Follow Up

Complications of surgical repair may include wound infection, CSF leak, meningitis, hydrocephalus, and retethering. These should be managed accordingly either by dural repair, VP shunt, or surgical exploration [20].

Patients may have decreased movement and weakness of the affected limb due to nerve root injury. In the long term, patients may develop spasticity, orthopedic problems and even poor school performance [22].

Patients with associated congenital malformation tend to have worse prognosis and require long term follow up for neurological deterioration [2].

Multiple Choice Questions

1. Cervical myelocystocele is a subtype of which spina bifida:
   - Common variant of open spinal dysraphisms
   - **Non common variant of closed spinal dysraphisms**
   - Non common variant of mixed spinal dysraphisms
   - Common variant of closed spinal dysraphisms
   - Common variant of mixed spinal dysraphisms
2. Cervical myelocystocele is usually linked to which vitamin deficiency:
   - Vitamin B1
   - Vitamin B2
   - Vitamin B3
   - Vitamin B6
   - **Vitamin B12**
3. Patients with cervical myelocystocele are:
   - Symptomless
   - Neurologically impaired
   - **Neurologically preserved**
   - Not indicated for surgery
   - Usually presenting with only pain
4. Modality of choice for the diagnosis of cervical myelocystocele is:
   - X-ray
   - US scan
   - CT scan
   - **MRI scan**
   - PET scan
5. Patients with cervical myelocystocele are usually treated with which of the following choices:
   - Watchful waiting
   - Conservative treatment

- **Surgical treatment**
- They don't need treatment unless neurological deficits occur
- They are emergency cases therefore they all need emergency treatment

6. Which of the following regarding cervical myelocystocele epidemiology is true:

- It's a disease that exclusively affects neonates
- It's a disease that has a huge incidence in the population
- **It's a disease with multifactorial risk factors**
- It's a disease that mainly happens due to vitamin B1 deficiency
- It's a disease that accounts for about 40% of neural tube defects

7. An important step that ensures the prevention of neurological deterioration in patients with cervical myelocystocele surgery is:

- Treating infections
- VP shunt
- Excision of the sac
- **Detethering of the cord**
- Cosmetic repair of the lesion

8. Cervical myelocystocele is strongly associated with which of the following:

- AV malformation
- Chiari I malformation
- **Chiari II malformation**
- Vertebral fractures
- Scoliosis

9. Surgery aims to prevent complications. Which of the following complications is most likely seen on follow up

- Ischemic infarction
- Radiculopathy
- **Paralyzed limbs**
- Bladder dysfunction
- Speech difficulties

10. Which of the following statements is true:

- On palpation, the skin is thin with a hair tuft
- **Associated congenital abnormalities are usually of bad prognosis**
- The lesion is seen as an open midline defect
- The defect has an X-linked type of inheritance
- Patients usually present late with neurological deficits

References

1. Meyer-Heim AD, Klein A, Boltshauser E. Cervical myelomeningocele—follow-up of five patients. Eur J Paediatr Neurol. 2003;7(6):407–12.
2. Klein O, Coulomb M-A, Ternier J, Lena G. Cervical myelocystocele: prenatal diagnosis and therapeutical considerations. Childs Nerv Syst. 2009;25(5):523–6.
3. McLone DG, Naidich TP. Terminal myelocystocele. Neurosurgery. 1985;16(1):36–43.
4. Salomão JF, Cavalheiro S, Matushita H, Leibinger RD, Bellas AR, Vanazzi E, et al. Cystic spinal dysraphism of the cervical and upper thoracic region. Childs Nerv Syst. 2006;22(3):234–42.
5. Pang D, Dias MS. Cervical myelomeningoceles. Neurosurgery. 1993;33(3):363–73.
6. Habibi Z, Nejat F, Tajik P, Kazmi SS, Kajbafzadeh A-M. Cervical myelomeningocele. Neurosurgery. 2006;58(6):1168–75.
7. van Gool JD, Hirche H, Lax H, De Schaepdrijver L. Folic acid and primary prevention of neural tube defects: a review. Reprod Toxicol. 2018;80:73–84.
8. Koc G, Doganay S, Dogan MS, Gorkem SB, Durmus NA. Non terminal myelocystocele of cervical region in a newborn. Eurorad. 2015. Available from: https://www.eurorad.org/case/13025.
9. Nishino A, Shirane R, So K, Arai H, Suzuki H, Sakurai Y. Cervical myelocystocele with Chiari II malformation: magnetic resonance imaging and surgical treatment. Surg Neurol. 1998;49(3):269–73.
10. Rossi A, Piatelli G, Gandolfo C, Pavanello M, Hoffmann C, Van Goethem JW, et al. Spectrum of nonterminal myelocystoceles. Neurosurgery. 2006;58(3):509–15.
11. Sauerbrei EE, Grant P. Prenatal diagnosis of myelocystoceles: report of two cases. J Ultrasound Med. 1999;18(3):247–52.
12. Shore RM, Chun RW, Strother CM. Lateral cervical meningocele. Clin Pediatr. 1982;21(7):430–3.
13. Noureldine MH, Peto I, Jallo GI, Agazzi S. Symptomatic recurrence of cervical spine myelomeningocele in an adult patient. World Neurosurg. 2020;137:376–8.
14. Jackson DL. Evaluation and management of pediatric neck masses: an otolaryngology perspective. Physician Assist Clin. 2018;3(2):245–69.
15. Andronikou S, Wieselthaler N, Fieggen AG. Cervical spina bifida cystica: MRI differentiation of the subtypes in children. Childs Nerv Syst. 2006;22(4):379–84.
16. Feltes CH, Fountas KN, Dimopoulos VG, Escurra AI, Boev A, Kapsalaki EZ, et al. Cervical meningocele in association with spinal abnormalities. Childs Nerv Syst. 2004;20(5):357–61.
17. Chandra RV, Kumar PM. Cervical myelocystocele: case report and review of literature. J Pediatr Neurosci. 2011;6(1):55–7.
18. Steinbok P. Dysraphic lesions of the cervical spinal cord. Neurosurg Clin N Am. 1995;6(2):367–76.
19. Armas-Melián K, Iglesias S, Ros B, Martínez-León MI, Arráez MÁ. Cervical myelomeningocele with CSF leakage: a case-based review. Childs Nerv Syst. 2020;36(11):2615–20.
20. Memet OM, Cinalli G, Maixner W. Spina bifida management and outcome. Milan: Springer; 2008.
21. Baaj AA. Handbook of spine surgery. Thieme; 2016.
22. Sun JCL, Steinbok P, Cochrane DD. Cervical myelocystoceles and meningoceles: long-term follow-up. Pediatr Neurosurg. 2000;33(3):118–22.
23. Raheja A, Gupta DK, Nalwa A, Suri V, Sharma BS. Non-terminal cervical myelocystocele: unusual cause of spastic quadriparesis in an adult. Neurol India. 2014;62(6):704–8.

Chapter 22
Congenital Spine Malformation in the Arab World

Sewar Elejla

Test your learning and check your understanding of this book's contents: use the "Springer Nature Flashcards" app to access questions using ▶ https://sn.pub/QCsfpd.
To use the app, please follow the instructions in Chap. 1.

22.1 Introduction

Inherited diseases genetically or in the acquired form will eventually alter the morphological pattern of an organ or particular part of the body. These types of malformations are caused without previous etiological factors "de-novo" or transmitted from parents, in both cases, the congenital anomaly will exist from the beginning of embryo life. On the other hand, disruptive anomalies are gained due to external factors such as infections, bleeding, and reduced blood flow, in which, the body's nature is developed normally but once affected by these factors, the affected part will be disrupted. Although the risk of recurrence for inherited disorders is different based on the mutations of the genes, it is very low in disruptive anomalies [1].

The exemplary conditions of the disruptive anomalies are hydran- and hemi-hydranencephaly [2], disruption of fetal brain FBD-like-phenotype [3], disruptive sequence of the twin [4].

S. Elejla (✉)
Al-Azhar University Gaza, Gaza, Palestine

K. F. AlAli, H. T. Hashim (eds.), *Congenital Spine Malformations*,
https://doi.org/10.1007/978-3-031-59031-3_22

22.2 Epidemiology

Of the congenital spinal malformations, neural tube defects (NTD) are one of the most common spinal malformations. The rates of NTD vary between countries and range from 0.62 to 13.8/1000 births [5]. The incidence of NTDs was reported to be high in Jordan which was estimated to be 1.1/1000 among 28,301 live births with male to female ratio of 1.2:1. Most NTDs in this study were myelomeningocele, followed by anencephaly [6].

National data from medical records in Oman reported an incidence of NTDs of 1.25 per 1000. The incidence of spinal Bifida was higher among newborns with increased maternal but not paternal age manifested as more affection in later-born children, especially with consanguinity marriages [7]. In Saudi Arabia, the incidence of anencephaly, spina bifida cystica, and encephalopathy were reported to be 0.43/1000, 0.33/1000, 0.08/1000 births, respectively [8]. In Sudan, the incidence of NTDs was reported to be 2.4/1000 live births and even higher at 3.48/1000 in two studies [9].

In many studies, female predominance was noticed in the incidence of NTD including myelomeningocele and anencephaly. The incidence of spinal malformations including NTDs is steadily and significantly decreasing in many Arab countries. This is largely attributed to the improved socioeconomic status, enhanced awareness of the risk of consanguinity marriages, and increased screening with the option of selective abortion in some countries after the proof of antenatal screening of NTDs [10].

22.3 Etiology and Pathogenesis

Most studies in the Arab world regarding congenital spinal malformation were about NTDs. NTDs are heterogenous conditions that result from failure of fusion of the neural tube in the midline during the embryogenic life in the 3–4 weeks of gestation. Therefore, many skeletal and muscular malformations in the structure that covers the neural abnormalities develop as a consequence of this. The most common three NTDs are three are anencephaly, spina bifida, and encephalocele.

Many etiologies play a role in the development of NTDs including race, place, socioeconomic status, education levels, nutrition, prenatal diagnosis, and screening programs in addition to the prophylactic programs such as folate administration in the country, presence of many predisposing factors such as the prevalence of consanguinity marriages, teratogens, and chromosomal abnormalities Family history and mother chronic disease have a role as well.

Another factor that was linked to the development of spinal malformations is heat exposure. For example, spina bifida and craniofacial defects were more common in Arab countries with high temperatures while some neural tube defects were less frequent in these countries [11]. However, this was in contrast to a previous study in Oman that showed that no environmental factors were associated with NTD and even high temperatures were excluded as a causative factor [7].

In a retrospective study in Sudan, like most countries in the world, spinal defects were more common than cranial defects with spina bifida being the commonest (73.2%) followed by encephaloceles (26.8%). The commonest site for spinal malformations was the lumbosacral region (34.6%). NTDs were especially common among younger mothers and consanguine parents. Around 25.4% of affected females reported infection during malaria, especially, malaria, based on this percentage, malaria or anti-malaria mediations were proposed as a possible etiology for NTDs as anti-malaria drugs are anti-folate drugs in their mechanism of action [12].

22.4 Prevention

As in other parts of the world, many Arab countries apply preventive programs for NTDs. These include the use of folic acid during pregnancy which was proven to be effective in reducing the incidence of NTD but also in preventing the recurrence. The recommended dose for those who already had previous NTDs is 4 mg of folic acid daily during the whole period of the pregnancy and 400 mg for those who do not have it [3]. In a study, only 12 countries in the Arab world fortify wheat with folic acid as a method to provide an adequate quantity of it for females at childhood age in an attempt to reduce the incidence of NTDs [5].

In most Arab countries, routine ultrasound scanning is done early in pregnancy for pregnant women at primary care centers in the first antenatal visit. In addition and to a less extent as an optional choice, many biochemical tests and maternal serum markers can be done in prenatal screening. These tests are usually followed, if there was any abnormality in the results, with further invasive tests such as amniocentesis. If these invasive tests showed to be abnormal, selective termination of the baby is allowed in some Arab countries not all of it. Such decisions have several legal, religious, social, and ethical implications.

Multidisciplinary teams are needed to manage these cases and to prevent their occurrence which includes the collaboration between antenatal clinics, genetic counseling, and fetal medicine teams.

Multiple Choice Questions

1. **The incidence of NTDs was reported to be high in ________ which was estimated to be 1.1/1000 among 28,301 live births.**

   A. Iraq
   B. Egypt
   C. Jordan
   D. Kuwait

2. **In _________, the incidence of NTDs was reported to be 2.4/1000 live births and even higher at 3.48/1000**.
   A. Sudan
   B. Saudi Arabia
   C. Palestine
   D. UAE

Answers
1. C
2. A

References

1. Al-Ghanim KA. Consanguineous marriage in the Arab societies. J Psychol Clin Psychiatry. 2020;11:166–8. https://doi.org/10.15406/jpcpy.2020.11.00692.
2. Arab world—total population 2011–2021. Statista. 2021. https://www.statista.com/statistics/806106/total-population-arab-league/#:~:text=Total%20population%20in%20the%20Arab%20world%202021&text=Therefore%2C%20the%20total%20population%20in. Retrieved 1 Nov 2022.
3. CDC. Folic acid. Centers for Disease Control and Prevention; 29 Oct 2018. https://www.cdc.gov/ncbddd/folicacid/about.html.
4. Consanguinity—an overview. 2021. https://www.sciencedirect.com/topics/medicine-and-dentistry/consanguinity#:~:text=The%20prevalence%20of%20congenital%20anomalies. Retrieved 1 Nov 2022.
5. Hamamy H. Epidemiological profile of neural tube defects in Arab countries. Middle East J Med Genet. 2014;3(1):1–10. https://doi.org/10.1097/01.mxe.0000438175.24428.e1.
6. Masri A. Neural tube defects in Jordan: a hospital based study. J Pediatr Neurol. 2015;4(4):245–9. https://doi.org/10.1055/s-0035-1557337.
7. Rajab A. Neural tube defects and congenital hydrocephalus in the Sultanate of Oman. J Trop Pediatr. 1998;44(5):300–3. https://doi.org/10.1093/tropej/44.5.300.
8. El-Awad ME-H, Sivasankaran S. Neural tube defects in southwestern region of Saudi Arabia. Ann Saudi Med. 1992;12(5):449–50. https://doi.org/10.5144/0256-4947.1992.449.
9. Salih MAM. Genetic disorders in Sudan. In: Genetic disorders among Arab populations. Springer; 2010. p. 575–612. https://doi.org/10.1007/978-3-642-05080-0_20.
10. Windham GC, Edmonds LD. Current trends in the incidence of neural tube defects. 2022. https://publications.aap.org/pediatrics/article-abstract/70/3/333/48526/Current-Trends-in-the-Incidence-of-Neural-Tube.
11. Haghighi M, Wright C, Ayer J, Urban M, Pham M, Boeckmann M, Areal A, Wernecke B, Swift C, Robinson M, Hetem R, Chersich M. Impacts of high environmental temperatures on congenital anomalies: a systematic review. Int J Environ Res Public Health. 2021;18(9):4910. https://doi.org/10.3390/ijerph18094910.
12. Sadik B, Babikir HE, Arbab MAR. Clinical profile of neural tube defects in Sudanese children: is malaria a risk factor? Sudanese J Paediatr. 2017;17(1):36–41. https://www.ncbi.nlm.nih.gov/pmc/articles/PMC5621856/.

Correction to: Tight Filum Terminale

Ahmad Rjoub, Motaz Daraghma, and Yazan Demaidi

Correction to:
Chapter 17 in: K. F. AlAli, H. T. Hashim (eds.), *Congenital Spine Malformations:* Clinical and Surgical Aspects, https://doi.org/10.1007/978-3-031-59031-3_17

This book was inadvertently published with an incorrect spelling of the author's name in Chapter 17 as Ahmed Rjoub. It has now been corrected to Ahmad Rjoub.

In addition to this, the affiliations of the below authors have been corrected to reflect their current affiliations as follows:

Motaz Daraghma, Faculty of Medicine, Arab American University of Palestine, Jenin, Palestine

Yazan Demaidi, Department of Medicine, An-Najah National University, Nablus, Palestine

The updated version of this book can be found at https://doi.org/10.1007/978-3-031-59031-3_17

K. F. AlAli, H. T. Hashim (eds.), *Congenital Spine Malformations*, https://doi.org/10.1007/978-3-031-59031-3_23

Index

K. F. AlAli, H. T. Hashim (eds.), *Congenital Spine Malformations*,
https://doi.org/10.1007/978-3-031-59031-3

MIX
Papier aus verantwortungsvollen Quellen
Paper from responsible sources
FSC® C105338

If you have any concerns about our products,
you can contact us on
ProductSafety@springernature.com

In case Publisher is established outside the EU,
the EU authorized representative is:
Springer Nature Customer Service Center GmbH
Europaplatz 3, 69115 Heidelberg, Germany

Printed by Libri Plureos GmbH
in Hamburg, Germany